Prostate Cancer
SOURCEBOOK

Health Reference Series

First Edition

Prostate Cancer
SOURCEBOOK

*Basic Consumer Health Information about
Prostate Cancer, Including Information about
the Associated Risk Factors, Detection, Diagnosis,
and Treatment of Prostate Cancer*

*Along with Information on Non-Malignant
Prostate Conditions, and Featuring a Section
Listing Support and Treatment Centers and a
Glossary of Related Terms*

Edited by
Dawn D. Matthews

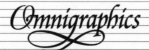

615 Griswold Street • Detroit, MI 48226

Bibliographic Note

Because this page cannot legibly accommodate all the copyright notices, the Bibliographic Note portion of the Preface constitutes an extension of the copyright notice.

Each new volume of the *Health Reference Series* is individually titled and called a "First Edition." Subsequent updates will carry sequential edition numbers. To help avoid confusion and to provide maximum flexibility in our ability to respond to informational needs, the practice of consecutively numbering each volume has been discontinued.

Edited by Dawn D. Matthews

Health Reference Series

Karen Bellenir, *Managing Editor*
David A. Cooke, MD, *Medical Consultant*
Maria Franklin, *Permissions Assistant*
Joan Margeson, *Research Associate*
Dawn Matthews, *Verification Assistant*
Carol Munson, *Permissions Assistant*
Jenifer Swanson, *Research Associate*

Omnigraphics, Inc.

Matthew P. Barbour, *Vice President, Operations*
Laurie Lanzen Harris, *Vice President, Editorial Director*
Kevin Hayes, *Production Coordinator*
Thomas J. Murphy, *Vice President, Finance and Controller*
Peter E. Ruffner, *Senior Vice President*
Jane J. Steele, *Marketing Coordinator*

Frederick G. Ruffner, Jr., *Publisher*

© 2001, Omnigraphics, Inc.

Library of Congress Cataloging-in-Publication Data

Prostate cancer sourcebook : basic consumer health information about prostate cancer, including information about the associated risk factors, detection, diagnosis, and treatment of prostate cancer; along with information on non-malignant prostate conditions, and featuring a section listing support and treatment centers and a glossary of related terms / edited by Dawn D. Matthews.-- 1st Ed.
  p. cm. -- (Health reference series)
Includes bibliographical references and index.
ISBN 0-7808-0324-8
  1. Prostate--Cancer. 2. Consumer education. I. Matthews, Dawn D. II. Series.

RC280.P7 P7599 2001
616.99'463--dc21

2001036360

∞

This book is printed on acid-free paper meeting the ANSI Z39.48 Standard. The infinity symbol that appears above indicates that the paper in this book meets that standard.

Printed in the United States

Table of Contents

Part III: Treatment of Prostate Cancer

Part IV: Non-Malignant Prostate Conditions and Related Concerns

Part V: Current Research Initiatives and Clinical Trials

Part VI: Additional Help and Information

Preface

About This Book

Approximately 16% of American men will be diagnosed with prostate cancer in their lifetime. Eight percent will develop significant symptoms and three percent will die of the disease. In the past prostate cancer was often not detected until a patient had symptoms of the disease, and treatment methods were often accompanied by undesirable side effects, such as impotence and incontinence. With newer screening methods, such as the Prostate-Specific-Antigen (PSA) test, prostate cancer can be—and usually is—diagnosed in the early, curable stage and treated with fewer side effects.

Prostate Cancer Sourcebook provides valuable information to those who have been diagnosed with prostate cancer, to individuals seeking information about screening and early detection, and to family members and loved ones of patients with prostate cancer. It describes the symptoms of prostate cancer, risk factors, diagnosis, and available treatment options. It includes information about non-malignant prostate disorders and offers section with resources for further help and information.

How to Use This Book

This book is divided into parts and chapters. Parts focus on broad areas of interest. Chapters are devoted to single topics within a part.

Part I: Cancer in Men includes an overview of men's cancer concerns, the top five cancers in men, and racial and ethnic prostate cancer patterns.

Part II: Introduction to Prostate Cancer provides basic facts about prostate cancer and its development, including screening tests for prostate cancer, signs and symptoms, and risk factors. A chapter describing how the urinary system works is included to help readers understand important anatomical issues related to the development of malignant and non-malignant prostate disease.

Part III: Treatment of Prostate Cancer contains information about understanding and choosing among the types of treatment for localized prostate cancer and disease that has spread. It also discusses post-treatment concerns, including infertility, impotence, and incontinence.

Part IV: Non-Malignant Prostate Conditions and Related Concerns explains conditions of the prostate that are non-cancerous. Men concerned about such disorders as prostatitis, impotence, and benign prostatic hyperplasia and their implications regarding cancer risk will find related information in this section.

Part V: Current Research Initiatives and Clinical Trials gives information about recent prostate cancer studies, taking part in clinical trials for prostate cancer, and newly developed treatment technologies.

Part VI: Additional Help and Information includes a glossary of important terms, a list of organizations serving people with prostate cancer, and a chapter on managing insurance issues.

Bibliographic Note

This volume contains documents and excerpts from publications issued by the following government agencies: National Cancer Institute (NCI); and National Institute of Diabetes and Digestive and Kidney Diseases (NIDDK).

In addition, this volume contains copyrighted articles from InteliHealth, Inc.; Omnigraphics; and the University of Iowa.

Full citation information is provided on the first page of each chapter. Every effort has been made to secure all necessary rights to reprint the copyrighted material. If any omissions have been made, please contact Omnigraphics to make corrections for future editions.

Acknowledgements

Thanks to Karen Bellenir for her guidance, to Dr. David Cooke for his help, and to Maria Franklin and Carol Munson for their work on this book.

Note from the Editor

This book is part of Omnigraphics' *Health Reference Series*. The series provides basic information about a broad range of medical concerns. It is not intended to serve as a tool for diagnosing illness, in prescribing treatments, or as a substitute for the physician/patient relationship. All persons concerned about medical symptoms or the possibility of disease are encouraged to seek professional care from an appropriate health care provider.

Our Advisory Board

The *Health Reference Series* is reviewed by an Advisory Board comprised of librarians from public, academic, and medical libraries. We would like to thank the following board members for providing guidance to the development of this series:

Dr. Lynda Baker, Associate Professor of Library and Information Science, Wayne State University, Detroit, MI

Nancy Bulgarelli, William Beaumont Hospital Library, Royal Oak, MI

Karen Imarasio, Bloomfield Township Public Library, Bloomfield Township, MI

Karen Morgan, Mardigian Library, University of Michigan-Dearborn, Dearborn, MI

Rosemary Orlando, St. Clair Shores Public Library, St. Clair Shores, MI

Medical Consultant

Medical consultation services are provided to the *Health Reference Series* editors by David A. Cooke, MD. Dr. Cooke is a graduate of Brandeis University, and he received his M.D. degree from the University of Michigan. He completed residency training at the University of Wisconsin Hospital and Clinics. He is board-certified in Internal

Medicine. Dr. Cooke currently works as part of the University of Michigan Health System and practices in Brighton, MI. In his free time, he enjoys writing, science fiction, and spending time with his family.

Health Reference Series *Update Policy*

The inaugural book in the *Health Reference Series* was the first edition of *Cancer Sourcebook* published in 1990. Since then, the Series has been enthusiastically received by librarians and in the medical community. In order to maintain the standard of providing high-quality health information for the layperson the editorial staff at Omnigraphics felt it was necessary to implement a policy of updating volumes when warranted.

Medical researchers have been making tremendous strides, and it is the purpose of the *Health Reference Series* to stay current with the most recent advances. Each decision to update a volume will be made on an individual basis. Some of the considerations will include how much new information is available and the feedback we receive from people who use the books. If there is a topic you would like to see added to the update list, or an area of medical concern you feel has not been adequately addressed, please write to:

Editor
Health Reference Series
Omnigraphics, Inc.
615 Griswold
Detroit, MI 48226

The commitment to providing on-going coverage of important medical developments has also led to some format changes in the *Health Reference Series*. Each new volume on a topic is individually titled and called a "First Edition." Subsequent updates will carry sequential edition numbers. To help avoid confusion and to provide maximum flexibility in our ability to respond to informational needs, the practice of consecutively numbering each volume has been discontinued.

Part One

Cancer in Men

Chapter 1

Cancer: An Overview

Introduction

This chapter contains important information about cancer. It describes some possible causes of cancer and mentions some ways to reduce the chance of getting the disease. It also tells about screening and early detection, symptoms, diagnosis, and treatment of cancer. Several sections of this chapter provide information to help people with cancer and their families cope with the disease.

Research has led to progress against many types of cancer—better treatments, a lower chance of death from the disease, and improved quality of life. Through research, knowledge about cancer keeps increasing. Scientists are learning more about what causes cancer and are finding new ways to prevent, detect, diagnose, and treat this disease.

What Is Cancer?

Cancer is a group of many related diseases that begin in cells, the body's basic unit of life. To understand cancer, it is helpful to know what happens when normal cells become cancerous. The body is made up of many types of cells. Normally, cells grow and divide to produce more cells only when the body needs them. This orderly process helps

Excerpted from "What You Need to Know about Cancer," National Cancer Institute, National Institute of Health (NIH), Publication Number 00-1566, 2000.

keep the body healthy. Sometimes, however, cells keep dividing when new cells are not needed. These extra cells form a mass of tissue, called a growth or tumor.

Tumors can be benign or malignant.

- *Benign tumors* are not cancer. They can often be removed and, in most cases, they do not come back. Cells from benign tumors do not spread to other parts of the body. Most important, benign tumors are rarely a threat to life.

- *Malignant tumors* are cancer. Cells in these tumors are abnormal and divide without control or order. They can invade and damage nearby tissues and organs. Also, cancer cells can break away from a malignant tumor and enter the bloodstream or the lymphatic system. That is how cancer spreads from the original cancer site to form new tumors in other organs. The spread of cancer is called metastasis.

Leukemia and lymphoma are cancers that arise in blood-forming cells. The abnormal cells circulate in the bloodstream and lymphatic system. They may also invade (infiltrate) body organs and form tumors.

Most cancers are named for the organ or type of cell in which they begin. For example, cancer that begins in the lung is lung cancer, and cancer that begins in cells in the skin known as melanocytes is called melanoma.

When cancer spreads (metastasizes), cancer cells are often found in nearby or regional lymph nodes (sometimes called lymph glands). If the cancer has reached these nodes, it means that cancer cells may have spread to other organs, such as the liver, bones, or brain. When cancer spreads from its original location to another part of the body, the new tumor has the same kind of abnormal cells and the same name as the primary tumor. For example, if lung cancer spreads to the brain, the cancer cells in the brain are actually lung cancer cells. The disease is called metastatic lung cancer (it is not brain cancer).

Possible Causes and Prevention of Cancer

The more we can learn about what causes cancer, the more likely we are to find ways to prevent it. In the laboratory, scientists explore possible causes of cancer and try to determine exactly what happens

4

in cells when they become cancerous. Researchers also study patterns of cancer in the population to look for risk factors, conditions that increase the chance that cancer might occur. They also look for protective factors, things that decrease the risk.

Even though doctors can seldom explain why one person gets cancer and another does not, it is clear that cancer is not caused by an injury, such as a bump or bruise. And although being infected with certain viruses may increase the risk of some types of cancer, cancer is not contagious; no one can "catch" cancer from another person.

Cancer develops over time. It is a result of a complex mix of factors related to lifestyle, heredity, and environment. A number of factors that increase a person's chance of developing cancer have been identified. Many types of cancer are related to the use of tobacco, what people eat and drink, exposure to ultraviolet (UV) radiation from the sun, and, to a lesser extent, exposure to cancer-causing agents (carcinogens) in the environment and the workplace. Some people are more sensitive than others to factors that can cause cancer.

Still, most people who get cancer have none of the known risk factors. And most people who do have risk factors do not get the disease.

Some cancer risk factors can be avoided. Others, such as inherited factors, are unavoidable, but it may be helpful to be aware of them. People can help protect themselves by avoiding known risk factors whenever possible. They can also talk with their doctor about regular checkups and about whether cancer screening tests could be of benefit.

These are some of the factors that increase the likelihood of cancer:

Tobacco

Smoking tobacco, using smokeless tobacco, and being regularly exposed to environmental tobacco smoke are responsible for one-third of all cancer deaths in the United States each year. Tobacco use is the most preventable cause of death in this country.

Smoking accounts for more than 85 percent of all lung cancer deaths. For smokers, the risk of getting lung cancer increases with the amount of tobacco smoked each day, the number of years they have smoked, the type of tobacco product, and how deeply they inhale. Overall, for those who smoke one pack a day, the chance of getting lung cancer is about 10 times greater than for nonsmokers. Cigarette smokers are also more likely than nonsmokers to develop several other types of cancer, including oral cancer and cancers of the larynx, esophagus, pancreas, bladder, kidney, and cervix. Smoking may also increase the likelihood of developing cancers of the stomach, liver, prostate, colon, and rectum. The risk of cancer begins to decrease soon after a smoker quits, and the risk continues to decline gradually each year after quitting.

People who smoke cigars or pipes have a risk for cancers of the oral cavity that is similar to the risk for people who smoke cigarettes. Cigar smokers also have an increased chance of developing cancers of the lung, larynx, esophagus, and pancreas.

The use of smokeless tobacco (chewing tobacco and snuff) causes cancer of the mouth and throat. Precancerous conditions, tissue changes that may lead to cancer, often begin to go away after a person stops using smokeless tobacco.

Studies suggest that exposure to environmental tobacco smoke, also called secondhand smoke, increases the risk of lung cancer for nonsmokers.

People who use tobacco in any form and need help quitting may want to talk with their doctor, dentist, or other health professional, or join a smoking cessation group sponsored by a local hospital or voluntary organization.

Diet

Researchers are exploring how dietary factors play a role in the development of cancer. Some evidence suggests a link between a high-fat diet and certain cancers, such as cancers of the colon, uterus, and prostate. Being seriously overweight may be linked to breast cancer among older women and to cancers of the prostate, pancreas, uterus, colon, and ovary. On the other hand, some studies suggest that foods containing fiber and certain nutrients may help protect against some types of cancer.

People may be able to reduce their cancer risk by making healthy food choices. A well-balanced diet includes generous amounts of foods that are high in fiber, vitamins, and minerals, and low in fat. This includes eating lots of fruits and vegetables and more whole-grain breads and cereals every day, fewer eggs, and not as much high-fat meat, high-fat dairy products (such as whole milk, butter, and most cheeses), salad dressing, margarine, and cooking oil.

Most scientists think that making healthy food choices is more beneficial than taking vitamin and mineral supplements.

Ultraviolet (UV) Radiation

UV radiation from the sun causes premature aging of the skin and skin damage that can lead to skin cancer. Artificial sources of UV radiation, such as sunlamps and tanning booths, also can cause skin damage and probably an increased risk of skin cancer. To help reduce the risk of skin cancer caused by UV radiation, it is best to reduce exposure to the midday sun (from 10 a.m. to 3 p.m.). Another simple rule is to avoid the sun when your shadow is shorter than you are.

Wearing a broad-brimmed hat, UV-absorbing sunglasses, long pants, and long sleeves offers protection. Many doctors believe that in addition to avoiding the sun and wearing protective clothing, wearing a sunscreen (especially one that reflects, absorbs, and/or scatters both types of ultraviolet radiation) may help prevent some forms of skin cancer. Sunscreens are rated in strength according to a sun protection factor (SPF). The higher the SPF, the more sunburn protection is provided. Sunscreens with an SPF of 12 through 29 are adequate for most people, but sunscreens are not a substitute for avoiding the sun and wearing protective clothing.

Alcohol

Heavy drinkers have an increased risk of cancers of the mouth, throat, esophagus, larynx, and liver. (People who smoke cigarettes and drink heavily have an especially high risk of getting these cancers.) Some studies suggest that even moderate drinking may slightly increase the risk of breast cancer.

Ionizing Radiation

Cells may be damaged by ionizing radiation from x-ray procedures, radioactive substances, rays that enter the Earth's atmosphere from outer space, and other sources. In very high doses, ionizing radiation may cause cancer and other diseases. Studies of survivors of the atomic bomb in Japan show that ionizing radiation increases the risk of developing leukemia and cancers of the breast, thyroid, lung, stomach, and other organs.

Before 1950, x-rays were used to treat noncancerous conditions (such as an enlarged thymus, enlarged tonsils and adenoids, ringworm of the scalp, and acne) in children and young adults. Those who have received radiation therapy to the head and neck have a higher-than-average risk of developing thyroid cancer years later. People with a history of such treatments should report it to their doctor.

Radiation that patients receive as therapy for cancer can also damage normal cells. Patients may want to talk with their doctor about the effect of radiation treatment on their risk of a second cancer. This risk can depend on the patient's age at the time of treatment as well as on the part of the body that was treated.

X-rays used for diagnosis expose people to lower levels of radiation than x-rays used for therapy. The benefits nearly always outweigh the risks. However, repeated exposure could be harmful, so it is a good idea for people to talk with their doctor about the need for each x-ray and to ask about the use of shields to protect other parts of the body.

Chemicals and Other Substances

Being exposed to substances such as certain chemicals, metals, or pesticides can increase the risk of cancer. Asbestos, nickel, cadmium, uranium, radon, vinyl chloride, benzidene, and benzene are examples of well-known carcinogens. These may act alone or along with another carcinogen, such as cigarette smoke, to increase the risk of cancer. For example, inhaling asbestos fibers increases the risk of lung diseases, including cancer, and the cancer risk is especially high for asbestos workers who smoke. It is important to follow work and safety rules to avoid or minimize contact with dangerous materials.

Diethylstilbestrol (DES)

DES is a synthetic form of estrogen that was used between the early 1940s and 1971. Some women took DES during pregnancy to prevent certain complications.

There is evidence that DES-exposed sons may have testicular abnormalities, such as undescended or abnormally small testicles. The possible risk for testicular cancer in these men is under study.

Close Relatives with Certain Types of Cancer

Some types of cancer (including melanoma and cancers of the breast, ovary, prostate, and colon) tend to occur more often in some families than in the rest of the population. It is often unclear whether a pattern of cancer in a family is primarily due to heredity, factors in the family's environment or lifestyle, or just a matter of chance.

Researchers have learned that cancer is caused by changes (called mutations or alterations) in genes that control normal cell growth and cell death. Most cancer-causing gene changes are the result of factors in lifestyle or the environment. However, some alterations that may lead to cancer are inherited; that is, they are passed from parent to child. But having such an inherited gene alteration does not mean that the person is certain to develop cancer; it means that the risk of cancer is increased.

Screening and Early Detection

Sometimes, cancer can be found before the disease causes symptoms. Checking for cancer (or for conditions that may lead to cancer) in a person who does not have any symptoms of the disease is called screening.

In routine physical exams, the doctor looks for anything unusual and feels for any lumps or growths. Specific screening tests, such as lab tests, x-rays, or other procedures, are used routinely for only a few types of cancer.

Colon and Rectum

A number of screening tests are used to find colon and rectal (colorectal) cancer. If a person is over the age of 50 years, has a family medical history of colorectal cancer, or has any other risk factors for colorectal cancer, a doctor may suggest one or more of these tests. Sometimes tumors in the colon or rectum can bleed. The fecal occult blood test checks for small amounts of blood in the stool.

The doctor sometimes uses a thin, lighted tube called a sigmoidoscope to examine the rectum and lower colon. Or, to examine the entire colon and rectum, a lighted instrument called a colonoscope is used. If abnormal areas are seen, tissue can be removed and examined under a microscope.

A barium enema is a series of x-rays of the colon and rectum. The patient is given an enema with a solution that contains barium, which outlines the colon and rectum on the x-rays. A digital rectal exam is an exam in which the doctor inserts a lubricated, gloved finger into the rectum to feel for abnormal areas.

Although it is not certain that screening for other cancers actually saves lives, doctors also may suggest screening for cancers of the skin, lung, and oral cavity. And doctors may offer to screen men for prostate or testicular cancer.

Doctors consider many factors before recommending a screening test. They weigh factors related to the individual, the test, and the cancer that the test is intended to detect. For example, doctors take into account the person's age, medical history and general health, family history, and lifestyle. The doctor pays special attention to a person's risk for developing specific types of cancer. In addition, the doctor will assess the accuracy and the risks of the screening test and any followup tests that may be necessary. Doctors also consider the effectiveness and side effects of the treatment that will be needed if cancer is found.

People may want to discuss any concerns or questions they have about screening with their doctors, so they can weigh the pros and cons and make informed decisions about having screening tests.

Symptoms of Cancer

Cancer can cause a variety of symptoms. These are some of them:

- Thickening or lump in the breast or any other part of the body
- Obvious change in a wart or mole
- A sore that does not heal
- Nagging cough or hoarseness
- Changes in bowel or bladder habits
- Indigestion or difficulty swallowing
- Unexplained changes in weight
- Unusual bleeding or discharge

When these or other symptoms occur, they are not always caused by cancer. They may also be caused by infections, benign tumors, or other problems. It is important to see the doctor about any of these symptoms or about other physical changes. Only a doctor can make a diagnosis. One should not wait to feel pain. Early cancer usually does not cause pain.

Diagnosis

If symptoms are present, the doctor asks about the person's medical history and performs a physical exam. In addition to checking general signs of health, the doctor may order various tests and exams. These may include laboratory tests and imaging procedures. A biopsy is usually necessary to determine whether cancer is present.

Laboratory Tests

Blood and urine tests can give the doctor important information about a person's health. In some cases, special tests are used to measure the amount of certain substances, called tumor markers, in the blood, urine, or certain tissues. Tumor marker levels may be abnormal if certain types of cancer are present. However, lab tests alone cannot be used to diagnose cancer.

Imaging

Images (pictures) of areas inside the body help the doctor see whether a tumor is present. These pictures can be made in several ways.

X-rays are the most common way to view organs and bones inside the body. A computed tomography (CT or CAT) scan is a special kind of imaging that uses a computer linked to an x-ray machine to make a series of pictures.

In radionuclide scanning, the patient swallows or receives an injection of a radioactive substance. A machine (scanner) measures radioactivity levels in certain organs and prints a picture on paper or film. The doctor can detect abnormal areas by looking at the amount of radioactivity in the organs. The radioactive substance is quickly eliminated by the patient's body after the test is done.

Ultrasonography is another procedure for viewing areas inside the body. High-frequency sound waves that cannot be heard by humans enter the body and bounce back. Their echoes produce a picture called a sonogram. These pictures are shown on a monitor like a TV screen and can be printed on paper.

In MRI, a powerful magnet linked to a computer is used to make detailed pictures of areas in the body. These pictures are viewed on a monitor and can also be printed.

Biopsy

A biopsy is almost always necessary to help the doctor make a diagnosis of cancer. In a biopsy, tissue is removed for examination under a microscope by a pathologist. Tissue may be removed in three ways: endoscopy, needle biopsy, or surgical biopsy.

- During an endoscopy, the doctor can look at areas inside the body through a thin, lighted tube. Endoscopy allows the doctor to see what's going on inside the body, take pictures, and remove tissue or cells for examination, if necessary.

- In a needle biopsy, the doctor takes a small tissue sample by inserting a needle into the abnormal (suspicious) area.

- A surgical biopsy may be excisional or incisional. In an excisional biopsy, the surgeon removes the entire tumor, often with some surrounding normal tissue. In an incisional biopsy, the doctor removes just a portion of the tumor. If cancer is present, the entire tumor may be removed immediately or during another operation.

Patients sometimes worry that having a biopsy (or any other type of surgery for cancer) will spread the disease. This is a very rare occurrence. Surgeons use special techniques and take many precautions to prevent cancer from spreading during surgery. For example, if tissue samples must be removed from more than one site, they use different instruments for each one. Also, a margin of normal tissue is often removed along with the tumor. Such efforts reduce the chance that cancer cells will spread into healthy tissue.

Some people may be concerned that exposing cancer to air during surgery will cause the disease to spread. This is not true. Exposure to air does not cause the cancer to spread.

Patients should discuss their concerns about the biopsy or other surgery with their doctor.

Staging

When cancer is diagnosed, the doctor will want to learn the stage, or extent, of the disease. Staging is a careful attempt to find out whether the cancer has spread and, if so, to which parts of the body. Treatment decisions depend on the results of staging. The doctor may order more laboratory tests and imaging studies or additional biopsies to find out whether the cancer has spread. An operation called a laparotomy can help the doctor find out whether cancer has spread within the abdomen. During this operation, a surgeon makes an incision into the abdomen and removes samples of tissue.

Handling the Diagnosis

It is natural for anyone facing cancer to be concerned about what the future holds. Understanding the nature of cancer and what to expect can help patients and their loved ones plan treatment, anticipate lifestyle changes, and make financial decisions. Cancer patients frequently ask their doctor or search on their own for statistics to answer the question, "What is my prognosis?"

Prognosis is a prediction of the future course and outcome of a disease, and an indication of the likelihood of recovery from that disease. However, it is only a prediction. When doctors discuss a patient's prognosis, they are attempting to project what is likely to occur for that individual patient. A cancer patient's prognosis can be affected by many factors, particularly the type of cancer, the stage of the disease, and its grade (how closely the cancer resembles normal tissue and how fast the cancer is likely to grow and spread). Other factors that may also affect the prognosis include the patient's age, general health, and response to treatment. As these factors change over time, a patient's prognosis is also likely to change.

Sometimes people use statistics to try to figure out their chances of being cured. However, for individual patients and their families, statistics are seldom helpful because they reflect the experience of a large group of patients. Statistics cannot predict what will happen to a particular patient because no two patients are alike; treatment and responses vary greatly.

If people want prognostic information, they should talk with the doctor. The doctor who is most familiar with a person's situation is in the best position to help interpret statistics and discuss prognosis. But even the doctor may not be able to describe exactly what to expect.

Seeking information about prognosis and statistics can help some people reduce their fears. How much information to seek and how to deal with it are personal matters.

Treatment

Treatment for cancer depends on the type of cancer; the size, location, and stage of the disease; the person's general health; and other factors. The doctor develops a treatment plan to fit each person's situation.

People with cancer are often treated by a team of specialists, which may include a surgeon, radiation oncologist, medical oncologist, and others. Most cancers are treated with surgery, radiation therapy, chemotherapy, hormone therapy, or biological therapy. The doctors may decide to use one treatment method or a combination of methods.

Clinical trials (research studies) offer important treatment options for many people with cancer. Research studies evaluate promising new therapies and answer scientific questions. The goal of such trials is to find treatments that are more effective in controlling cancer with fewer side effects.

Getting a Second Opinion

Before starting treatment, the patient may want to have a second opinion from another doctor about the diagnosis and the treatment plan. Some insurance companies require a second opinion; others may cover a second opinion if the patient requests it.

There are a number of ways to find a doctor who can give a second opinion:

- The patient's doctor may be able to suggest specialists to consult.

- The Cancer Information Service, at 1-800-4-CANCER, can tell callers about cancer treatment facilities all over the country, including cancer centers and other programs supported by the National Cancer Institute (NCI).

- Patients can get the names of doctors from their local medical society, a nearby hospital, or a medical school.

- The Official ABMS Directory of Board Certified Medical Specialists lists doctors names along with their specialty and their educational background. This resource, produced by the American Board of Medical Specialties (ABMS), is available in most public libraries.

Preparing for Treatment

Many people with cancer want to take an active part in decisions about their medical care. They want to learn all they can about their disease and their treatment choices. However, the shock and stress that people often feel after a diagnosis of cancer can make it hard for them to think of everything they want to ask the doctor. Often it is helpful to prepare a list of questions in advance. To help remember what the doctor says, patients may take notes or ask whether they may use a tape recorder. Some people also want to have a family member or friend with them when they talk to the doctor—to take part in the discussion, to take notes, or just to listen.

These are some questions a patient may want to ask the doctor before treatment begins:

- What is my diagnosis?

- Is there any evidence the cancer has spread? What is the stage of the disease?

- What are my treatment choices? Which do you recommend for me? Why?

- What new treatments are being studied? Would a clinical trial be appropriate for me?

- What are the expected benefits of each kind of treatment?

- What are the risks and possible side effects of each treatment?

- Is infertility a side effect of cancer treatment? Can anything be done about it?

- What can I do to prepare for treatment?

- How often will I have treatments?

- How long will treatment last?

- Will I have to change my normal activities? If so, for how long?

- What is the treatment likely to cost?

Patients do not need to ask all their questions or remember all the answers at one time. They will have many chances to ask the doctor to explain things and to get more information.

Methods of Treatment and Their Side Effects

Treatment for cancer can be either local or systemic. Local treatments affect cancer cells in the tumor and the area near it. Systemic treatments travel through the bloodstream, reaching cancer cells all over the body. Surgery and radiation therapy are types of local treatment. Chemotherapy, hormone therapy, and biological therapy are examples of systemic treatment.

It is hard to protect healthy cells from the harmful effects of cancer treatment. Because treatment does damage healthy cells and tissues, it often causes side effects. The side effects of cancer treatment depend mainly on the type and extent of the treatment. Also, the effects may not be the same for each person, and they may change for a person from one treatment to the next. A patient's reaction to treatment is closely monitored by physical exams, blood tests, and other tests. Doctors and nurses can explain the possible side effects of treatment, and they can suggest ways to reduce or eliminate problems that may occur during and after treatment.

Surgery is therapy to remove the cancer; the surgeon may also remove some of the surrounding tissue and lymph nodes near the tumor. Sometimes surgery is done on an outpatient basis, or the patient may have to stay in the hospital. This decision depends mainly on the type of surgery and the type of anesthesia.

The side effects of surgery depend on many factors, including the size and location of the tumor, the type of operation, and the patient's general health. Although patients are often uncomfortable during the first few days after surgery, this pain can be controlled with medicine. Patients should feel free to discuss ways of relieving pain with the doctor or nurse. It is also common for patients to feel tired or weak for a while after surgery. The length of time it takes to recover from an operation varies among patients.

Radiation therapy (also called radiotherapy) uses high-energy rays to kill cancer cells. For some types of cancer, radiation therapy may be used instead of surgery as the primary treatment. Radiation therapy also may be given before surgery (neoadjuvant therapy) to shrink a tumor so that it is easier to remove. In other cases, radiation therapy is given after surgery (adjuvant therapy) to destroy any cancer cells that may remain in the area. Radiation also may be used alone, or along with other types of treatment, to relieve pain or other problems if the tumor cannot be removed. Radiation therapy can be in either of two forms: external or internal. Some patients receive both.

External radiation comes from a machine that aims the rays at a specific area of the body. Most often, this treatment is given on an outpatient basis in a hospital or clinic. There is no radioactivity left in the body after the treatment.

With internal radiation (also called implant radiation, interstitial radiation, or brachytherapy), the radiation comes from radioactive material that is sealed in needles, seeds, wires, or catheters and placed directly in or near the tumor. Patients may stay in the hospital while the level of radiation is highest. They may not be able to have visitors during the hospital stay or may have visitors for only a short time. The implant may be permanent or temporary. The amount of radiation in a permanent implant goes down to a safe level before the person leaves the hospital. The doctor will advise the patient if any special precautions should be taken at home. With a temporary implant, there is no radioactivity left in the body after the implant is removed.

The side effects of radiation therapy depend on the treatment dose and the part of the body that is treated. Patients are likely to become extremely tired during radiation therapy, especially in the later weeks of treatment. Extra rest is often necessary, but doctors usually encourage patients to try to stay as active as they can between rest periods.

With external radiation, there may be permanent darkening or "bronzing" of the skin in the treated area. In addition, it is common to have temporary hair loss in the treated area and for the skin to become red, dry, tender, and itchy. Radiation therapy also may cause a decrease in the number of white blood cells, cells that help protect the body against infection.

Although radiation therapy can cause side effects, these can usually be treated or controlled. Most side effects are temporary, but some may be persistent or occur months to years later.

Chemotherapy is the use of drugs to kill cancer cells. The doctor may use one drug or a combination of drugs. Chemotherapy may be the only kind of treatment a patient needs, or it may be combined with other forms of treatment. Neoadjuvant chemotherapy refers to drugs given before surgery to shrink a tumor; adjuvant chemotherapy refers to drugs given after surgery to help prevent the cancer from recurring. Chemotherapy also may be used (alone or along with other forms of treatment) to relieve symptoms of the disease.

Chemotherapy is usually given in cycles: a treatment period (one or more days when treatment is given) followed by a recovery period (several days or weeks), then another treatment period, and so on. Most anticancer drugs are given by injection into a vein (IV); some are injected into a muscle or under the skin; and some are given by mouth.

Often, patients who need many doses of IV chemotherapy receive the drugs through a catheter (a thin, flexible tube) that stays in place until treatment is over. One end of the catheter is placed in a large vein in the arm or the chest; the other end remains outside the body. Anticancer drugs are given through the catheter. Patients who have catheters avoid the discomfort of having a needle inserted into a vein for each treatment. Patients and their families learn how to care for the catheter and keep it clean.

Sometimes the anticancer drugs are given in other ways. For example, in an approach called intraperitoneal chemotherapy, anticancer drugs are placed directly into the abdomen through a catheter. To reach cancer cells in the central nervous system (CNS), the patient may receive intrathecal chemotherapy. In this type of treatment, the anticancer drugs enter the cerebrospinal fluid through a needle placed in the spinal column or a device placed under the scalp.

Usually a patient has chemotherapy as an outpatient (at the hospital, at the doctor's office, or at home). However, depending on which drugs are given, the dose, how they are given, and the patient's general health, a short hospital stay may be needed.

The side effects of chemotherapy depend mainly on the drugs and the doses the patient receives. As with other types of treatment, side effects vary from person to person. Generally, anticancer drugs affect cells that divide rapidly. In addition to cancer cells, these include blood cells, which fight infection, help the blood to clot, and carry oxygen to all parts of the body. When blood cells are affected, patients are more likely to get infections, may bruise or bleed easily, and may feel unusually weak and very tired. Rapidly dividing cells in hair roots and cells that line the digestive tract may also be affected. As a result, side effects may include loss of hair, poor appetite, nausea and vomiting, diarrhea, or mouth and lip sores.

Hair loss is a major concern for many people with cancer. Some anticancer drugs only cause the hair to thin, while others may result in the loss of all body hair. Patients may cope better if they prepare for hair loss before starting treatment (for example, by buying a wig or hat). Most side effects go away gradually during the recovery periods between treatments, and hair grows back after treatment is over.

Some anticancer drugs can cause long-term side effects such as loss of fertility (the ability to produce children). Loss of fertility may be temporary or permanent, depending on the drugs used and the patient's age and sex. For men, sperm banking before treatment may be an option. Women's menstrual periods may stop, and they may have hot flashes and vaginal dryness. Periods are more likely to return in young women.

Hormone therapy is used against certain cancers that depend on hormones for their growth. Hormone therapy keeps cancer cells from getting or using the hormones they need. This treatment may include the use of drugs that stop the production of certain hormones or that change the way they work. Another type of hormone therapy is surgery to remove organs (such as the ovaries or testicles) that make hormones.

Hormone therapy can cause a number of side effects. Patients may feel tired, have fluid retention, weight gain, hot flashes, nausea and vomiting, changes in appetite, and, in some cases, blood clots. In women, hormone therapy may cause interrupted menstrual periods and vaginal dryness. Hormone therapy in women may also cause either a loss of or an increase in fertility; women taking hormone therapy should talk with their doctor about contraception during treatment.

In men, hormone therapy may cause impotence, loss of sexual desire, or loss of fertility. Depending on the drug used, these changes may be temporary, long lasting, or permanent. Patients may want to talk with their doctor about these and other side effects.

Biological therapy (also called immunotherapy) helps the body's natural ability (immune system) to fight disease or protects the body from some of the side effects of cancer treatment. Monoclonal antibodies, interferon, interleukin-2, and colony-stimulating factors are some types of biological therapy.

The side effects caused by biological therapy vary with the specific treatment. In general, these treatments tend to cause flu-like symptoms, such as chills, fever, muscle aches, weakness, loss of appetite, nausea, vomiting, and diarrhea. Patients also may bleed or bruise easily, get a skin rash, or have swelling. These problems can be severe, but they go away after the treatment stops.

Bone marrow transplantation (BMT) or peripheral stem cell transplantation (PSCT) may also be used in cancer treatment. The transplant may be autologous (the person's own cells that were saved earlier), allogeneic (cells donated by another person), or syngeneic (cells donated by an identical twin). Both BMT and PSCT provide the patient with healthy stem cells (very immature cells that mature into blood cells). These replace stem cells that have been damaged or destroyed by very high doses of chemotherapy and/or radiation treatment.

Patients who have a BMT or PSCT face an increased risk of infection, bleeding, and other side effects due to the high doses of chemotherapy and/or radiation they receive. The most common side effects associated with the transplant itself are nausea and vomiting during the transplant, and chills and fever during the first day or so. In addition, graft-versus-host disease (GVHD) may occur in patients who receive bone marrow from a donor. In GVHD, the donated marrow (the graft) reacts against the patient's (the host's) tissues (most often the liver, the skin, and the digestive tract).

GVHD can be mild or very severe. It can occur any time after the transplant (even years later). Drugs may be given to reduce the risk of GVHD and to treat the problem if it occurs.

Nutrition During Cancer Treatment

Eating well during cancer treatment means getting enough calories and protein to help prevent weight loss and maintain strength. Eating well often helps people feel better and have more energy. Some people with cancer find it hard to eat because they lose their appetite. In addition, common side effects of treatment, such as nausea, vomiting, or mouth and lip sores, can make eating difficult. Often, foods taste different. Also, people being treated for cancer may not feel like eating when they are uncomfortable or tired.

Doctors, nurses, and dietitians can offer advice on how to get enough calories and protein during cancer treatment.

Pain Control

Pain is a common problem for people with some types of cancer, especially when the cancer grows and presses against other organs and nerves. Pain may also be a side effect of treatment. However, pain can generally be relieved or reduced with prescription medicines or over-the-counter drugs as recommended by the doctor. Other ways to reduce pain, such as relaxation exercises, may also be useful. It is important for patients to report pain so that steps can be taken to help relieve it.

Rehabilitation

Rehabilitation is an important part of the overall cancer treatment process. The goal of rehabilitation is to improve a person's quality of life. The medical team, which may include doctors, nurses, a physical therapist, an occupational therapist, or a social worker, develops a rehabilitation plan to meet each patient's physical and emotional needs, helping the patient return to normal activities as soon as possible.

Patients and their families may need to work with an occupational therapist to overcome any difficulty in eating, dressing, bathing, using the toilet, or other activities. Physical therapy may be needed to regain strength in muscles and to prevent stiffness and swelling. Physical therapy may also be necessary if an arm or leg is weak or paralyzed, or if a patient has trouble with balance.

Followup Care

It is important for people who have had cancer to continue to have examinations regularly after their treatment is over. Followup care ensures that any changes in health are identified, and if the cancer recurs, it can be treated as soon as possible. Checkups may include a careful physical exam, imaging procedures, endoscopy, or lab tests.

Between scheduled appointments, people who have had cancer should report any health problems to their doctor as soon as they appear.

Support for People with Cancer

Living with a serious disease is not easy. People with cancer and those who care about them face many problems and challenges. Having helpful information and support services can make it easier to cope with these problems.

Friends and relatives can be very supportive. Also, it helps many patients to discuss their concerns with others who have cancer. People with cancer often get together in support groups, where they can share what they have learned about coping with their disease and the effects of their treatment. It is important to keep in mind, however, that each person is different. Treatments and ways of dealing with cancer that work for one person may not be right for another—even if they both have the same kind of cancer. It is always a good idea to discuss the advice of friends and family members with the doctor.

People living with cancer may worry about caring for their families, keeping their jobs, or continuing daily activities. Concerns about tests, treatments, hospital stays, and medical bills are also common. Doctors, nurses, and other members of the health care team can answer questions about treatment, working, or other activities. Meeting with a social worker, counselor, or member of the clergy can be helpful to people who want to talk about their feelings or discuss their concerns. Often, a social worker can suggest resources for help with rehabilitation, emotional support, financial aid, transportation, or home care.

Clinical Trials

Doctors all over the country conduct many types of clinical trials (research studies in which people take part voluntarily). These include studies of ways to prevent, detect, diagnose, and treat cancer; studies of the psychological effects of the disease; and studies of ways to improve comfort and quality of life.

People who take part in clinical trials have the first chance to benefit from new approaches. They also make important contributions to medical science. Although clinical trials may pose some risks, researchers take very careful steps to protect people who take part.

People who are interested in being part of a clinical trial should talk with their doctor.

National Cancer Institute Booklets

The National Cancer Institute (NCI) booklets and other materials are available from the Cancer Information Service by calling 1-800-4-CANCER. They are also available on the NCI Web site, which is located at http://cancer.gov/publications on the Internet.

Chapter 2

Top Five Cancers in Men

Five Most Common Cancers in Each Racial/Ethnic Group

The top five cancer age-adjusted incidence rates and mortality rates are displayed for men in each racial/ethnic group. Rankings for the total white population are identical to those for the non-Hispanic white population and are not shown in the following set of graphs. Among men, lung and bronchus, prostate and colorectal cancer appear among the top five cancer incidence rates in every racial/ethnic group.

Prostate cancer is the highest reported cancer among American Indian, black, Filipino, Japanese, non-Hispanic white and whites. Cancer of the lung and bronchus is highest among men in the remaining racial/ethnic groups.

Lung cancer is the leading cause of cancer death among men in all racial/ethnic groups except American Indians, who have higher mortality from cancers of the prostate, stomach and liver.

Cancer of the prostate or colon and rectum is the second leading cause of cancer death among men in most other racial/ethnic groups. The exception is Chinese men, for whom liver cancer ranks second in mortality.

Miller, B.A., Kolonel, L.N., Bernstein, L., Young, Jr., J.L., Swanson, G. M., West, D., Key, C.R., Liff, J.M., Glover, C.S., Alexander, G.A., et al. (eds). Excerpted from *Racial/Ethnic Patterns of Cancer in the United States 1988-1992;* National Cancer Institute (NCI); NIH Publication Number 96-4104. Bethesda, MD, 1996.

Table 2.1. Five Most Frequently Diagnosed Cancers Seer Incidence Rates for Men, 1988-1992 (Rates are "average annual" per 100,000 population, age-adjusted to 1970 U.S. standard), continued on next page.

Alaska Native

Lung and Bronchus	81.1
Colon and Rectum	79.7
Prostate	46.1
Stomach	27.2
Kidney and Renal Pelvis	19.0*

American Indian (New Mexico)

Prostate	52.5
Colon and Rectum	18.6
Kidney and Renal Pelvis	15.6
Lung and Bronchus	14.4
Liver & Intrahep.	13.1*

Black

Prostate	180.6
Lung and Bronchus 117.0	
Colon and Rectum	60.7
Oral Cavity	20.4
Stomach	17.9

Chinese

Lung and Bronchus	52.1
Prostate	46.0
Colon and Rectum	44.8
Liver & Intrahep.	20.8
Stomach	15.7

Filipino

Prostate	69.8
Lung and Bronchus	52.6
Colon and Rectum	35.4
Non-Hodgkin's Lymphoma	12.9
Liver & Intrahep.	10.5

Hawaiian

Lung and Bronchus	89.0
Prostate	57.2
Colon and Rectum	42.4
Stomach	20.5
Non-Hodgkin's Lymphoma	12.5

Table 2.1. Five Most Frequently Diagnosed Cancers Seer Incidence Rates for Men, 1988-1992 (Rates are "average annual" per 100,000 population, age-adjusted to 1970 U.S. standard), continued from previous page.

Japanese

Prostate	88.0
Colon and Rectum	64.1
Lung and Bronchus	43.0
Stomach	30.5
Urinary Bladder	13.7

Korean

Lung and Bronchus	53.2
Stomach	48.9
Colon and Rectum	31.7
Liver & Intrahep.	24.8
Prostate	24.2

Vietnamese

Lung and Bronchus	70.9
Liver & Intrahep.	41.8
Prostate	40.0
Colon and Rectum	30.5
Stomach	25.8

White Non-Hispanic

Prostate	137.9
Lung and Bronchus	79.0
Colon and Rectum	57.6
Urinary Bladder	33.1
Non-Hodgkin's Lymphoma	19.1

Hispanic (Total)

Prostate	89.0
Lung and Bronchus	41.8
Colon and Rectum	38.3
Urinary Bladder	15.8
Stomach	15.3

White Hispanic

Prostate	92.8
Lung and Bronchus	44.0
Colon and Rectum	40.2
Urinary Bladder	16.7
Stomach	16.2

* = Rate is based on fewer than 25 cases and may be subject to greater variability than the other rates which are based on larger numbers.

Table 2.2. Five Most Common Types of Cancer Deaths, United States Mortality Rates, 1988-1992. (Rates are "average annual" per 100,000 population, age-adjusted to 1970 U.S. standard), continued on next page.

Alaska Native

Lung and Bronchus	69.4
Colon and Rectum	27.2
Stomach	18.91*
Kidney and Renal Pelvis	13.4*
Nasopharynx	11.6*

American Indian (New Mexico)

Prostate	16.2
Stomach	11.2*
Liver & Intrahep.	11.2*
Lung and Bronchus	10.4*
Colon and Rectum	8.5*

Black

Lung and Bronchus	105.6
Prostate	53.7
Colon and Rectum	28.2
Esophagus	14.8
Pancreas	14.4

Chinese

Lung and Bronchus	40.1
Liver & Intrahep.	17.7
Colon and Rectum	15.7
Stomach	10.5
Pancreas	6.7

Filipino

Lung and Bronchus	29.8
Prostate	13.5
Colon and Rectum	11.4
Liver & Intrahep.	7.8
Leukemia	5.7

Table 2.2. Five Most Common Types of Cancer Deaths, United States Mortality Rates, 1988-1992. (Rates are "average annual" per 100,000 population, age-adjusted to 1970 U.S. standard), continued from previous page.

Hawaiian

Lung and Bronchus	88.9
Colon and Rectum	23.7
Prostate	19.9
Stomach	14.4
Pancreas	12.8

Japanese

Lung and Bronchus	32.4
Colon and Rectum	20.5
Stomach	17.4
Prostate	11.7
Pancreas	8.5

White Non-Hispanic

Lung and Bronchus	74.2
Prostate	24.4
Colon and Rectum	23.4
Pancreas	9.8
Leukemia	8.6

Hispanic (Total)

Lung and Bronchus	32.4
Prostate	15.3
Colon and Rectum	12.8
Stomach	8.4
Pancreas	7.1

White Hispanic

Lung and Bronchus	33.6
Prostate	15.9
Colon and Rectum	13.4
Stomach	8.8
Pancreas	7.4

* = Rate is based on fewer than 25 deaths and may be subject to greater variability than the other rates which are based on larger numbers.

Stomach cancer appears in the top five causes of cancer deaths among men in all groups except black, Filipinos and non-Hispanic whites. Cancer of the pancreas is among the top five causes of cancer deaths in men for all groups except Alaska Natives, American Indians and Filipinos.

Cancer of the Lung and Bronchus

Cancer of the lung and bronchus (hereafter, lung cancer) is the second most common cancer among men and is the leading cause of cancer death in men. Among men, aged-adjusted lung cancer incidence rates (per 100,000) range from a low of about 14 among American Indians to a high of 117 among blacks, and eight-fold difference. Between these two extremes, rates fall into two groups ranging from 42 to 53 for Hispanics, Japanese, Chinese, Filipinos, and Koreans and from 71 to 89 for Vietnamese, whites, Alaska Natives and Hawaiians.

In the 30-54 year age group, incidence rates among men are double those among women in most of the racial/ethnic groups. In white non-Hispanics and white Hispanics, however incidence rates for women are closer to those for men. This suggests that smoking cessation and prevention programs may have been especially successful among white men and/or that such programs have not been as effective among white women.

Age-adjusted mortality rates follow similar racial/ethnic patterns to those for the incidence rates. Among men, the incidence and mortality rates are very similar. Filipino men are an exception, with an incidence rate nearly twice as large as their mortality rate.

Cigarette smoking accounts for nearly 90% of all lung cancers. Passive smoking also contributes to the development of lung cancer among nonsmokers. Certain occupational exposures such as asbestos exposure are also known to cause lung cancer. Air pollution is a probably cause, but makes a relatively small contribution to incidence and mortality rates. In certain geographic areas of the United States, indoor exposure to radon may also make a small contribution to the total incidence of lung cancer.

Cancer of the Colon and Rectum

Cancers of the colon and rectum are the fourth most commonly diagnosed cancers and rank second among cancer deaths in the United States. The incidence rates show wide divergence by racial/ethnic group, with rates in the Alaska Native population that are over four times as high as rates in the American Indian population (New Mexico) for both men and women. There are only minor differences between men and women, in the order of incidence rates by racial/ethnic group. After Alaska Natives, the next highest rates in men are among Japanese, black and non-Hispanic white populations. These are followed by Chinese, Hawaiians and white Hispanics; and then Filipinos, Koreans and Vietnamese. Incidence rates for both men and women are substantially lower among American Indians in New Mexico (18.6 per 100,000 in men).

Although the pattern of incidence rates by race/ethnicity is similar for each sex, the ratio of male-to female rates varies. Among Filipinos and Japanese, men experience an excess of greater than 60% while among American Indians, Alaska Natives and Vietnamese the male excess is much lower at only 13-22%. It is interesting that, although the Alaska Natives have the highest colorectal cancer incidence rates of all groups and the American Indians experience the lowest, the gender ratios of these two native American groups are similar.

Mortality patterns by race/ethnicity for cancers of the colon and rectum are similar to those for incidence, with several notable exceptions. Black, Alaska Native, and white non-Hispanic men and women, as well as Hawaiian and Japanese men, have comparatively high mortality rates. The high mortality rates among Alaska Natives and Japanese men are consistent with the high incidence rates in these groups. However, the mortality rates among white non-Hispanic and black men and women, and among Hawaiian men, appear disproportionately high.

Colon cancer accounts for 59% (Korean men) to 81% (Alaska Native men) of the combined colon and rectum cancer incidence rates. This is reflected in a racial/ethnic pattern for colon cancer incidence rates that is quite similar to the pattern for both sites combined. Incidence and mortality rates for cancers of the colon and rectum increase with age. Interestingly, the incidence rate for Hawaiian men is highest in the 55-69 year age group, and their mortality rate is second only to black men in this age group.

Migrant and other studies have provided very strong evidence that colorectal cancer risk is modifiable, and that differences in population rates may therefore be explained by lifestyle or environmental factors. Dietary factors and exercise appear to be very important. Migrants to the United States (from Japan and other countries where rates of colon and rectal cancer are lower than in the U.S.) have higher rates than do those who remain in their native country. Studies have shown that first and second generation American offspring from these migrant groups develop these cancers at rates reaching or exceeding those of the United States white population.

Cancer of the Stomach

Stomach cancer was the most common form of cancer in the world in the 1970s and early 1980s, and is probably now only surpassed by lung cancer. Stomach cancer incidence rates show substantial variation internationally. Rates are highest in Japan and eastern Asia, but other areas of the world have high stomach cancer incidence rates including eastern Europe and parts of Latin America. Incidence rates are generally lower in western Europe and the United States. Stomach cancer incidence and mortality rates have been declining for several decades in most areas of the world. For one subsite of the stomach, the cardia, incidence rates appear to be increasing, particularly among white men.

Stomach cancer incidence rates for the racial/ethnic populations in the SEER regions can be grouped broadly into three levels. Those with high age-adjusted incidence rates are Koreans, Vietnamese, Japanese, Alaska Natives and Hawaiians. Those with intermediate incidence rates are white Hispanic, Chinese, and black populations. Filipinos and non-Hispanic whites have substantially lower incidence rates than the other groups. These patterns hold for both men and women when rates are available for both sexes.

The incidence rate for Korean men is 1.6 times the rate in Japanese men, the group with the second highest rate, and is 2.4 times the rate in Hawaiians. The range in incidence rates is narrower among the groups in the intermediate level. The incidence rate for Korean men is nearly 5.8 times greater than the rate in Filipino men, the group with the lowest incidence rate. The male-to-female ratio of age-adjusted incidence rates is highest for Koreans (2.6) and followed closely by non-Hispanic whites and blacks (2.5 and 2.4, respectively). The ratio is less than two for other racial-ethnic groups. Notably, the incidence rates for Vietnamese men and women are the same.

The racial/ethnic patterns of stomach cancer mortality in the United States are similar to those for incidence. These patterns remain when incidence and mortality rates are calculated for the three age groups. There are some differences in the ratios of incidence rates to mortality rates. Filipinos show relatively high ratios of incidence to mortality (greater than 2); Japanese, Alaska Natives, white Hispanics, Chinese, and non-Hispanic whites show intermediate ratios

(1.5-1.9); blacks and Hawaiians show low ratios of incidence to mortality rates (1.0-1.4).

Better techniques for food preservation and storage are often cited as reasons for the decline in stomach cancer incidence worldwide. Refrigeration has resulted in lower intake of salted, smoked and pickled foods and greater availability of fresh fruits and vegetables. Evidence is strong that salt intake is a major determinant of stomach cancer risk. Cigarette smoking may also play a role. Infection with helicobacter pylori, the major cause of chronic active gastritis, also appears to be important in the development of stomach cancer.

Cancer of the Liver and Intrahepatic Bile Ducts

Primary cancers of the liver and intrahepatic bile ducts are far more common in regions of Africa and Asia than in the United States, where they only account for about 1.5% of all cancer cases. Five-year survival rates are very low in the United States, usually less than 10%. Reported statistics for these cancers often include mortality rates that equal or exceed the incidence rates. This discrepancy (more deaths than cases) occurs when the cause of death is misclassified as "liver cancer" for some patients whose cancer originated as a primary cancer in another organ and spread (metastasized) to become a "secondary" cancer in the liver.

Non-Hispanic white men and women have the lowest age-adjusted incidence rates (SEER areas) and mortality rates (United States) for primary liver cancer. Rates in the black populations and Hispanic populations are roughly twice as high as the rates in whites. The highest incidence rate is in Vietnamese men (41.8 per 100,000), probably reflecting risks associated with the high prevalence of viral hepatitis infections in their homeland. Other Asian-American groups also have liver cancer incidence and mortality rates several times higher than the white population. Age-adjusted mortality rates among Chinese populations are the highest of all groups for which there are sufficient numbers to calculate rates. There were too few cases among Alaska Native and American Indian populations to calculate incidence or mortality rates. Most cases of liver cancer occur in the two older age groups, but younger adults are often affected in the high risk racial/ethnic groups.

About two-thirds of liver cancers are hepatocellular carcinomas (HCC), which is the cancer type most clearly associated with hepatitis B and Hepatitis C viral infections and cirrhosis. Certain molds that grow on stored foods are recognized risk factors in parts of Africa and

31

Asia. HCC occurs more frequently in men than in women by a ratio of two-to-one. About one-in-five liver cancers are cholangiocarcinomas, arising from branches of the bile ducts that are located within the liver. Certain liver parasites are recognized risk factors for this type of liver cancer, especially in parts of southeast Asia. Angiosarcomas are rare cancers that can arise from blood vessels within the liver. They account for about 1% of primary liver cancers and some of them have been associated with industrial exposures to vinyl chloride.

Non-Hodgkin's Lymphoma

Lymphomas, which include Hodgkin's disease and non-Hodgkin's lymphoma, are the fifth most common type of cancer diagnosed and the sixth most common cancer cause of death in the United States. Of the two basic lymphoma types, non-Hodgkin's lymphoma is the more common.

The age-adjusted incidence rates for non-Hodgkin's lymphoma are higher among men than women in every racial/ethnic group except Koreans, in which there is a slight preponderance among women. In both men and women, non-Hodgkin's lymphoma incidence rates are highest among non-Hispanic whites (19.1 and 12.0 per 100,000 men and women, respectively) and lowest among Koreans (5.8 and 6.0 per 100,000). This corresponds to a high to low ratio of the rates (white non-Hispanic to Korean) of 3.3 for men, and 2.0 for women.

Vietnamese men have the second highest rates (after whites), followed by white Hispanic, black, Filipino, Hawaiian, Chinese and Japanese men. There were too few cases diagnosed in Alaska Native and American Indian (New Mexico) men to calculate reliable rates.

Age adjusted mortality rates of non-Hodgkin's lymphoma are consistent with the incidence rates with one exception: the mortality rate for Hawaiian men (8.8 per 100,000) exceeds that of any other group, even though the corresponding incidence rate is considerably lower than that of white non-Hispanics. There are an insufficient number of deaths from non-Hodgkin's lymphoma among Hawaiian women to reliably assess the mortality rate for that group.

In every group, incidence rates increase with age, however the magnitude of this increase varies by racial/ethnic group. For example, from ages 30-54 years to ages 70 years and older, the incidence of non-Hodgkin's lymphoma increases about five-fold among white non-Hispanics, but 11-fold among Filipino men. Among women, the comparable rates increase eight-fold among white non-Hispanic men, but 16-fold among Filipinos. These differences reflect high incidence rates among older Filipinos, similar to those of white non-Hispanics. These high rates are not reflected, however, in the mortality data for Filipinos. Among those aged 30-54 years rates among black men and women are close to those among white non-Hispanics. Rates among black men and women aged 70 years and older, however, are only about one-half those of white non-Hispanics.

Cancer of the Kidney

Historically, incidence rates for kidney cancer hove included cancers of the renal cells (in the main part of the kidney) and the renal pelvis (the lower part of the kidney where urine collects before entering the ureter and continuing to the bladder), although there is evidence that these cancers have different characteristics. They are presented together here for continuity. About one of five kidney cancers occur in the renal pelvis. Internationally, the highest incidence rates occur in the United States, Canada, Northern Europe, Australia, and New Zealand. The lowest rates are in Thailand, China, and the Philippines. Rates in these countries are about one-third the rates in the high risk countries.

During the years 1988 to 1992, in the SEER regions, the incidence rates for kidney cancers are abut twice as high in men as in women. The highest rates in the SEER regions are in American Indian men in New Mexico. Rates are somewhat lower in blacks, Hispanics and white non-Hispanics (ranging from 10 to 13 per 100,000 for men and about six per 100,000 for women). The lowest incidence rates occur in the Asian populations. There were too few cases among Alaska Native and Vietnamese populations to calculate rates. Age-specific incidence rates for kidney cancer demonstrate a small, temporary peak in early childhood due to Wilm's tumor, an uncommon tumor of the kidney with a good prognosis. Rates then decline with age and remain low until they finally surpass the early peak at around age 40. The racial/ethnic patterns for ages 55-69 years and 70 years and over are similar to those for all ages combined. In the 30-54 year old age group, racial/ethnic differences are slight.

Kidney cancer has a relatively high mortality rate in all racial/ethnic populations. Following the incidence pattern, mortality rates are about twice as high in men as in women, regardless of age. There are too few deaths among American Indian (New Mexico), Alaska Native and Hawaiian populations to calculate reliable rates. Mortality rates for blacks are comparable to those for white non-Hispanics. Rates for the other races are lower. In all racial/ethnic groups the mortality rates increase with age.

Cancers of the kidney and renal pelvis share many risk factors although the strengths of the associations differ. For both types of cancer the only well-established risk factor is cigarette smoking. Compared to nonsmokers, smokers have about twice the risk for renal cell cancer and about four times the risk for renal pelvis cancer than nonsmokers. Other probable risk factors include obesity and, especially for cancer of the renal pelvis, heavy long-term use of analgesics (medications used to relieve pain). Cessation of cigarette smoking is the best single step in preventing these cancers. It is estimated that this measure alone would reduce by one-half the number of renal pelvis cancers and by one-third the number of renal cell cancers.

Cancer of the Urinary Bladder

The highest incidence rates for bladder cancer are found in industrialized countries such as the United States, Canada, France, Denmark, Italy, and Spain. Rates are lower in England, Scotland, and Eastern Europe. The lowest rates are in Asia and South America, where the incidence is only about 30% as high as in the United States. In all countries the rates are higher for men than women.

In the SEER regions, for the period 1988 to 1992, the incidence rates are generally three to four times higher in men than in women. Among men, the highest rates are in white non-Hispanics (33.1 per 100,000). The rates for black men and Hispanic men are similar and are about one-half the white non-Hispanic rate. The lowest rates are in the Asian populations.

The incidence of bladder cancer increases dramatically with age among men and women in all populations. Rates in those aged 70 years and older are approximately two to three times higher than those aged 5-69 years, and about 15 to 20 times higher than those aged 30-54 years.

Mortality rates are two to three times higher for men than women. While incidence rates in the white population exceed those for the black population, such is not the case for mortality where the rates are much closer together. This difference in survival between black and white populations reflects the fact that in whites a larger proportion of these cancers are diagnosed at an early more treatable stage. Mortality rates for Hispanic and Asian men and women are only about one-half those for whites and blacks.

Cigarette smoking is an established risk factor for urinary bladder cancer. It is estimated that about 50% of these cancers in men and 30% in women are due to smoking. Occupational exposures may account for up to 25% of all urinary bladder cancers. Most of the occupationally accrued risk is due to exposure to a group of chemicals known as arylamines. Occupations with high exposure to arylamines include dye workers, rubber workers, leather workers, truck drivers, painters, and aluminum workers. Because of this association with bladder cancer, some arylamines have been eliminated or greatly reduced in occupational settings. Coffee, alcohol, and artificial sweeteners have all been studied as risk factors for bladder cancer, but associations, if they exist, are weak. The greatest prevention strategy is reduction in the consumption of cigarettes. Cigarette use increases one's risk for bladder cancer by two to five times. When cigarette smokers quit, their risk declines in two to four years.

Cancer of the Oral Cavity

Cancer of the oral cavity includes the following subsites: lip (excluding skin of the lip), tongue, salivary glands, gum, mouth, pharynx, oropharynx, and hypopharynx.

For SEER areas, incidence rates for oral cavity cancer are two to four times higher among men than women for all racial/ethnic groups except Filipinos, among whom the rates for the tow sexes are similar. Two few cases occurred among Alaska Natives, American Indians, Koreans, and Vietnamese women for the calculation of reliable rates. Across racial/ethnic groups, the incidence rates vary by a factor of four in men and about three in women. Among men, the highest rates are in blacks, followed by whites (especially non-Hispanic whites), Vietnamese, and native Hawaiians.

Incidence rates for oral cavity cancer increase with age in all groups except the oldest age group of black men and women. The greatest increase in rates occurs between the 30-54 year old group and the 55-69 year old group. For several racial/ethnic and sex groups, the numbers of cases were too few to compute reliable rates by age category.

Mortality rates for oral cavity cancer are substantially lower than incidence rates, reflecting the reasonably high survival rates for this cancer site. The mortality rates increase with age in all groups except black men and women aged 70 years and older. Tobacco use, including pipes, cigars, cigarettes, and chewing tobacco are well-established causes of cancers of the oral cavity. Chewing of betel nut, not a common practice in the United States but a widespread habit in some parts of the world, is also a known cause. Alcohol consumption, especially when combined with cigarette smoking, is an established risk factor. Both factors together interact synergistically. Finally, some evidence suggests that diets high in fruits and vegetables reduce the risk of developing this cancer.

Chapter 3

Racial/Ethnic Prostate Cancer Patterns in the United States

Prostate cancer is the leading cancer diagnosed among men in the United States. However, racial/ethnic variations in the SEER data are striking: the incidence rate among black men (180.6 per 100,000) is more than seven times that among Koreans (24.2). Indeed, blacks in the U.S. have the highest rates of this cancer in the world. Although the incidence among whites is quite high, it is distinctly lower than among blacks. Asian and native American men have the lowest rates. The very low rate in Korean men probably reflects the fact that most of the Koreans in the SEER areas are recent immigrants from Asia, where rates are lower than in the United States.

Age-specific incidence rates show dramatic increases between age categories. The remarkably sharp increase in incidence with age is a hallmark of this cancer. Sixty percent of all newly diagnosed prostate cancer cases and almost 80% of all deaths occur in men 70 years of age and older. Mortality rates for prostate cancer are much lower than the incidence rates, because survival for men with this cancer is generally quite high.

Prostate cancer incidence has been increasing rapidly in recent years. Most of this increase has been attributed to the greater use of

Miller, B.A., Kolonel, L.N., Bernstein, L., Young, Jr., J.L., Swanson, G. M., West, D., Key, C.R., Liff, J.M., Glover, C.S., Alexander, G.A., et al. (eds). Excerpted from *Racial/Ethnic Patterns of Cancer in the United States 1988-1992;* National Cancer Institute (NCI); NIH Publication Number 96-4104. Bethesda, MD, 1996.

screening modalities, and especially the widespread introduction of the prostate-specific antigen (PSA) test. The causes of prostate cancer are not known. Men with a family history of prostate cancer are at increased risk, but whether this is genetic or due to shared environmental influences, or both, is not known. It is thought that whatever the causal factors are, they act by altering the balance of male hormones in the body. Some research has suggested that diets high in fat and red meats increase risk, while a high intake of fruits and vegetables may offer some protection. There is current interest in the possibility that the low risk of prostate cancer in certain Asian populations may result from their high intake of soy products.

Table 3.1. SEER Incidence Rates of Prostate Cancer among Men, 1988-1992

Alaska Native	46.1
American Indian (New Mexico)	52.5
Black	180.6
Chinese	46.0
Filipino	69.8
Hawaiian	57.2
Japanese	88.0
Korean	24.2
Vietnamese	40.0
White	134.7
Hispanic (Total)	89.0
White Hispanic	92.8
White Non-Hispanic	137.9

Table 3.2. United States Prostate Cancer MORTALITY Rates Among Men, 1988-1992

Alaska Native	*
American Indian (New Mexico)	16.2
Black	53.7
Chinese	6.6
Filipino	13.5
Hawaiian	19.9
Japanese	11.7
Korean	N/A
Vietnamese	N/A
White	24.1
Hispanic (Total)	15.3
White Hispanic	15.9
White Non-Hispanic	24.4

Rates are "average annual" per 100,000 population, age-adjusted to 1970 U.S. standard; N/A = information not available; * = rate not calculated when fewer than 25 cases.

Table 3.3. Seer Prostate Cancer Incidence Rates Among Men By Age At Diagnosis, 1988-1992.

Age 30-54

Alaska Native	*
American Indian (New Mexico)	*
Black	19.3
Chinese	*
Filipino	*
Hawaiian	*
Japanese	*
Korean	*
Vietnamese	*
White	12.4
Hispanic (Total)	7.0
White Hispanic	7.3
White Non-Hispanic	3.1

Age 55-69

Alaska Native	*
American Indian (New Mexico)	131.7
Black	576.4
Chinese	105.7
Filipino	151.7
Hawaiian	143.1
Japanese	203.1
Korean	*
Vietnamese	*
White	395.8
Hispanic (Total)	242.8
White Hispanic	251.2
White Non-Hispanic	409.1

Age 70+

Alaska Native	*
American Indian (New Mexico)	524.7
Black	1594.2
Chinese	504.2
Filipino	770.2
Hawaiian	575.6
Japanese	957.8
Korean	275.9
Vietnamese	402.7
White	1264.8
Hispanic (Total)	878.0
White Hispanic	918.9
White Non-Hispanic	1284.3

Rates Are Per 100,000 Population, Age-Adjusted To 1970 U.S. Standard; * = Rate Not Calculated When Fewer Than 25 Cases.

Table 3.4. United States Prostate Cancer MORTALITY Rates Among Men by Age at Death, 1988-1992.

Age 30-54

Alaska Native	*
American Indian (New Mexico)	*
Black	2.9
Chinese	*
Filipino	*
Hawaiian	*
Japanese	*
Korean	N/A
Vietnamese	N/A
White	0.9
Hispanic (Total)	0.7
White Hispanic	0.7
White Non-Hispanic	1.0

Age 55-69

Alaska Native	*
American Indian (New Mexico)	*
Black	100.4
Chinese	6.2
Filipino	9.4
Hawaiian	*
Japanese	12.9
Korean	N/A
Vietnamese	N/A
White	36.6
Hispanic (Total)	23.9
White Hispanic	24.7
White Non-Hispanic	37.2

Age 70+

Alaska Native	*
American Indian (New Mexico)	218.6
Black	625.6
Chinese	90.7
Filipino	189.5
Hawaiian	251.8
Japanese	156.6
Korean	N/A
Vietnamese	N/A
White	298.2
Hispanic (Total)	188.8
White Hispanic	195.4
White Non-Hispanic	302.0

Rates Are "Average Annual" Per 100,000 Population, Age-Adjusted To 1970 U.S. Standard; N/A = Data Unavailable; * = Fewer Than 25 Deaths.

Chapter 4

Metastatic Cancer

The chapter contains a series of questions and answers regarding metastatic cancer, and will be helpful to individuals seeking information on this aspect of cancer.

What is cancer?

Cancer is a group of many related diseases that begin in cells, the body's basic unit of life. The body is made up of many types of cells. Normally, cells grow and divide to produce more cells only when the body needs them. This orderly process helps keep the body healthy. Sometimes cells keep dividing when new cells are not needed. These extra cells may form a mass of tissue, called a growth or tumor. Tumors can be either benign (not cancerous) or malignant (cancerous).

Cancer can begin in any organ or tissue of the body. The original tumor is called the primary cancer or primary tumor and is usually named for the part of the body in which it begins.

What is metastasis?

Metastasis means the spread of cancer. Cancer cells can break away from a primary tumor and travel through the bloodstream or lymphatic system to other parts of the body.

From CancerNet, "Questions and Answers about Metastatic Cancer," National Cancer Institute (NCI), 2000.

Cancer cells may spread to lymph nodes near the primary tumor (regional lymph nodes). This is called nodal involvement, positive nodes, or regional disease. Cancer cells can also spread to other parts of the body, distant from the primary tumor. Doctors use the term metastatic disease or distant disease to describe cancer that spreads to other organs or to lymph nodes other than those near the primary tumor.

When cancer cells spread and form a new tumor, the new tumor is called a secondary, or metastatic, tumor. The cancer cells that form the secondary tumor are like those in the original tumor. That means, for example, that if breast cancer spreads (metastasizes) to the lung, the secondary tumor is made up of abnormal breast cells (not abnormal lung cells). The disease in the lung is metastatic breast cancer (not lung cancer).

Is it possible to have a metastasis without having a primary cancer?

No. A metastasis is a tumor that started from a cancer cell or cells in another part of the body. Sometimes, however, a primary cancer is discovered only after a metastasis causes symptoms. For example, a man whose prostate cancer has spread to the bones in the pelvis may have lower back pain (caused by the cancer in his bones) before experiencing any symptoms from the prostate tumor itself.

How does a doctor know whether a cancer is a primary or a secondary tumor?

The cells in a metastatic tumor resemble those in the primary tumor. Once the cancerous tissue is examined under a microscope to determine the cell type, a doctor can usually tell whether that type of cell is normally found in the part of the body from which the tissue sample was taken. For instance, breast cancer cells look the same whether they are found in the breast or have spread to another part of the body. So, if a tissue sample taken from a tumor in the lung contains cells that look like breast cells, the doctor determines that the lung tumor is a secondary tumor.

Metastatic cancers may be found at the same time as the primary tumor, or months or years later. When a second tumor is found in a patient who has been treated for cancer in the past, it is more often a metastasis than another primary tumor.

In a small number of cancer patients, a secondary tumor is diagnosed, but no primary cancer can be found, in spite of extensive tests.

Doctors refer to the primary tumor as unknown or occult, and the patient is said to have cancer of unknown primary origin (CUP).

What treatments are used for metastatic cancer?

When cancer has metastasized, it may be treated with chemotherapy, radiation therapy, biological therapy, hormone therapy, surgery, or a combination of these. The choice of treatment generally depends on the type of primary cancer, the size and location of the metastasis, the patient's age and general health, and the types of treatments used previously. In patients diagnosed with CUP, it is still possible to treat the disease even when the primary tumor cannot be located.

New cancer treatments are currently under study. To develop new treatments, the National Cancer Institute (NCI) sponsors clinical trials (research studies) with cancer patients in many hospitals, universities, medical schools, and cancer centers around the country. Clinical trials are a critical step in the improvement of treatment. Before any new treatment can be recommended for general use, doctors conduct studies to find out whether the treatment is both safe for patients and effective against the disease. The results of such studies have led to progress not only in the treatment of cancer, but in the detection, diagnosis, and prevention of the disease as well. Patients interested in participating in research should ask their doctor to find out whether they are eligible for a clinical trial.

Part Two

Introduction to
Prostate Cancer

Chapter 5

Prostate Cancer: An Overview

Introduction

This chapter contains important information about cancer of the prostate. Prostate cancer is the most common type of cancer in men in the United States (other than skin cancer). Of all the men who are diagnosed with cancer each year, more than one-fourth have prostate cancer.

This chapter mentions some possible causes of prostate cancer. It also describes symptoms, diagnosis, treatment, and followup care. It has information to help men with prostate cancer and their families cope with the disease.

Research is increasing our understanding of prostate cancer. Scientists are learning more about the possible causes of prostate cancer and are looking for new ways to prevent, detect, diagnose, and treat this disease. Because of this research, men with prostate cancer now have a lower chance of dying from the disease.

The Prostate

The prostate is a gland in a man's reproductive system. It makes and stores seminal fluid, a milky fluid that nourishes sperm. This fluid is released to form part of semen.

The prostate is about the size of a walnut. It is located below the bladder and in front of the rectum. It surrounds the upper part of the

Excerpted from NIH Publication No. 00-1576, 2000.

49

urethra, the tube that empties urine from the bladder. If the prostate grows too large, the flow of urine can be slowed or stopped.

To work properly, the prostate needs male hormones (androgens). Male hormones are responsible for male sex characteristics. The main male hormone is testosterone, which is made mainly by the testicles. Some male hormones are produced in small amounts by the adrenal glands.

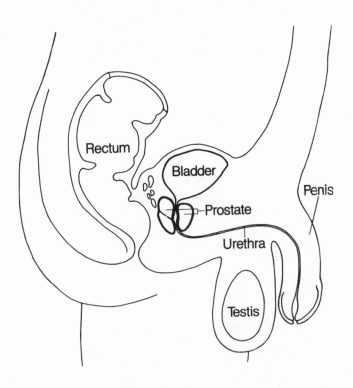

Figure 5.1. This picture shows the prostate and nearby organs.

Understanding the Cancer Process

Cancer is a group of many related diseases. These diseases begin in cells, the body's basic unit of life. Cells have many important functions throughout the body.

Normally, cells grow and divide to form new cells in an orderly way. They perform their functions for a while, and then they die. This process helps keep the body healthy.

Sometimes, however, cells do not die. Instead, they keep dividing and creating new cells that the body does not need. They form a mass of tissue, called a growth or tumor.

Tumors can be benign or malignant:

- **Benign** tumors are not cancer. They can usually be removed, and in most cases, they do not come back. Cells from benign tumors do not spread to other parts of the body. Most important, benign tumors of the prostate are not a threat to life.

  Benign prostatic hyperplasia (BPH) is the abnormal growth of benign prostate cells. In BPH, the prostate grows larger and presses against the urethra and bladder, interfering with the normal flow of urine. More than half of the men in the United States between the ages of 60 and 70 and as many as 90 percent between the ages of 70 and 90 have symptoms of BPH. For some men, the symptoms may be severe enough to require treatment.

- **Malignant** tumors are cancer. Cells in these tumors are abnormal. They divide without control or order, and they do not die. They can invade and damage nearby tissues and organs. Also, cancer cells can break away from a malignant tumor and enter the bloodstream and lymphatic system. This is how cancer spreads from the original (primary) cancer site to form new (secondary) tumors in other organs. The spread of cancer is called metastasis.

  When prostate cancer spreads (metastasizes) outside the prostate, cancer cells are often found in nearby lymph nodes. If the cancer has reached these nodes, it means that cancer cells may have spread to other parts of the body—other lymph nodes and other organs, such as the bones, bladder, or rectum. When cancer spreads from its original location to another part of the body, the new tumor has the same kind of abnormal cells and the same name as the primary tumor. For example, if prostate cancer spreads to the bones, the cancer cells in the new tumor are prostate cancer cells. The disease is metastatic prostate cancer; it is not bone cancer.

Prostate Cancer: Who's at Risk

The causes of prostate cancer are not well understood. Doctors cannot explain why one man gets prostate cancer and another does not.

Researchers are studying factors that may increase the risk of this disease. Studies have found that the following risk factors are associated with prostate cancer:

- *Age.* In the United States, prostate cancer is found mainly in men over age 55. The average age of patients at the time of diagnosis is 70.

- *Family history of prostate cancer.* A man's risk for developing prostate cancer is higher if his father or brother has had the disease.

- *Race.* This disease is much more common in African American men than in white men. It is less common in Asian and American Indian men.

- *Diet and dietary factors.* Some evidence suggests that a diet high in animal fat may increase the risk of prostate cancer and a diet high in fruits and vegetables may decrease the risk. Studies are in progress to learn whether men can reduce their risk of prostate cancer by taking certain dietary supplements.

Although a few studies suggested that having a vasectomy might increase a man's risk for prostate cancer, most studies do not support this finding. Scientists have studied whether benign prostatic hyperplasia, obesity, lack of exercise, smoking, radiation exposure, or a sexually transmitted virus might increase the risk for prostate cancer. At this time, there is little evidence that these factors contribute to an increased risk.

Detecting Prostate Cancer

A man who has any of the risk factors may want to ask a doctor whether to begin screening for prostate cancer (even though he does not have any symptoms), what tests to have, and how often to have them. The doctor may suggest either of the tests described below. These tests are used to detect prostate abnormalities, but they cannot show whether abnormalities are cancer or another, less serious condition. The doctor will take the results into account in deciding whether to check the patient further for signs of cancer. The doctor can explain more about each test.

- *Digital rectal exam*—the doctor inserts a lubricated, gloved finger into the rectum and feels the prostate through the rectal wall to check for hard or lumpy areas.

- *Blood test for prostate-specific antigen (PSA)*—a lab measures the levels of PSA in a blood sample. The level of PSA may rise in men who have prostate cancer, BPH, or infection in the prostate.

Recognizing Symptoms

Early prostate cancer often does not cause symptoms. But prostate cancer can cause any of these problems:

- A need to urinate frequently, especially at night;
- Difficulty starting urination or holding back urine;
- Inability to urinate;
- Weak or interrupted flow of urine;
- Painful or burning urination;
- Difficulty in having an erection;
- Painful ejaculation;
- Blood in urine or semen; or
- Frequent pain or stiffness in the lower back, hips, or upper thighs.

Any of these symptoms may be caused by cancer or by other, less serious health problems, such as BPH or an infection. A man who has symptoms like these should see his doctor or a urologist (a doctor who specializes in treating diseases of the genitourinary system).

Diagnosing Prostate Cancer

If a man has symptoms or test results that suggest prostate cancer, his doctor asks about his personal and family medical history, performs a physical exam, and may order laboratory tests. The exams and tests may include a digital rectal exam, a urine test to check for blood or infection, and a blood test to measure PSA. In some cases, the doctor also may check the level of prostatic acid phosphatase (PAP) in the blood, especially if the results of the PSA indicate there might be a problem.

The doctor may order exams to learn more about the cause of the symptoms. These may include:

- *Transrectal ultrasonography* — sound waves that cannot be heard by humans (ultrasound) are sent out by a probe inserted into the rectum. The waves bounce off the prostate, and a computer uses the echoes to create a picture called a sonogram.

- *Intravenous pyelogram* — a series of x-rays of the organs of the urinary tract.

- *Cystoscopy* — a procedure in which a doctor looks into the urethra and bladder through a thin, lighted tube.

Biopsy

If test results suggest that cancer may be present, the man will need to have a biopsy. During a biopsy, the doctor removes tissue samples from the prostate, usually with a needle. A pathologist looks at the tissue under a microscope to check for cancer cells. If cancer is present, the pathologist usually reports the grade of the tumor. The grade tells how much the tumor tissue differs from normal prostate tissue and suggests how fast the tumor is likely to grow. One way of grading prostate cancer, called the Gleason system, uses scores of 2 to 10. Another system uses G1 through G4. Tumors with higher scores or grades are more likely to grow and spread than tumors with lower scores.

A man who needs a biopsy may want to ask the doctor some of the following questions:

- How long will the procedure take? Will I be awake? Will it hurt?

- Are there any risks? What are the chances of infection or bleeding after the biopsy?

- How soon will I know the results?

- If I do have cancer, who will talk to me about treatment? When?

If the physical exam and test results do not suggest cancer, the doctor may recommend medicine to reduce the symptoms caused by an enlarged prostate. Surgery is another way to relieve these symptoms. The surgery most often used in such cases is called transurethral resection of the prostate (TURP or TUR). In TURP, an instrument is inserted through the urethra to remove prostate tissue that is pressing against the upper part of the urethra and restricting the flow of urine. (Patients may want to ask whether other procedures might be appropriate.)

Stages of Prostate Cancer

If cancer is found in the prostate, the doctor needs to know the stage, or extent, of the disease. Staging is a careful attempt to find out whether the cancer has spread and, if so, what parts of the body are affected. The doctor may use various blood and imaging tests to learn the stage of the disease. Treatment decisions depend on these findings.

Prostate cancer staging is a complex process. The doctor may describe the stage using a Roman number (I-IV) or a capital letter (A-D). These are the main features of each stage:

- *Stage I or Stage A*—The cancer cannot be felt during a rectal exam. It may be found by accident when surgery is done for another reason, usually for BPH. There is no evidence that the cancer has spread outside the prostate.

- *Stage II or Stage B*—The tumor involves more tissue within the prostate, it can be felt during a rectal exam, or it is found with a biopsy that is done because of a high PSA level. There is no evidence that the cancer has spread outside the prostate.

- *Stage III or Stage C*—The cancer has spread outside the prostate to nearby tissues.

- *Stage IV or Stage D*—The cancer has spread to lymph nodes or to other parts of the body.

Treatment for Prostate Cancer

Getting a Second Opinion

Decisions about prostate cancer treatment involve many factors. Before making a decision, a man may want to get a second opinion by asking another doctor to review the diagnosis and treatment options. A short delay will not reduce the chance that treatment will be successful. Some health insurance companies require a second opinion; many others will cover a second opinion if the patient requests it. There are a number of ways to find a doctor who can give a second opinion:

- The patient's doctor may be able to recommend a specialist or team of specialists to consult. Doctors who treat prostate cancer are urologists, radiation oncologists, and medical oncologists. Patients may find it helpful to talk to a specialist in each of these areas. Different types of specialists may have different thoughts about how best to manage prostate cancer.

- The Cancer Information Service, at 1-800-4-CANCER, can tell callers about treatment facilities, including cancer centers and other programs supported by the National Cancer Institute.

- People can get the names of doctors from their local medical society, a nearby hospital, or a medical school.

- The Official ABMS Directory of Board Certified Medical Specialists lists doctors' names along with their specialty and their educational background. This resource, produced by the American Board of Medical Specialties (ABMS), is available in most public libraries. The ABMS also has an online service that lists many board-certified physicians (http://www.certifieddoctor.org).

Preparing for Treatment

The doctor develops a treatment plan to fit each man's needs. Treatment for prostate cancer depends on the stage of the disease and the grade of the tumor (which indicates how abnormal the cells look, and how likely they are to grow or spread). Other important factors in planning treatment are the man's age and general health and his feelings about the treatments and their possible side effects.

Many men with prostate cancer want to learn all they can about their disease, their treatment choices, and the possible side effects of treatment, so they can take an active part in decisions about their medical care. Prostate cancer can be managed in a number of ways (with watchful waiting, surgery, radiation therapy, and hormonal therapy). If the doctor recommends watchful waiting, the man's health will be monitored closely, and he will be treated only if symptoms occur or worsen. Patients considering surgery, radiation therapy, or hormonal therapy may want to consult doctors who specialize in these types of treatment.

The patient and his doctor may want to consider both the benefits and possible side effects of each option, especially the effects on sexual activity and urination, and other concerns about quality of life.

These are some questions a patient may want to ask the doctor before treatment begins:

- What is the stage of the disease?
- What is the grade of the disease?
- What are my treatment choices? Is watchful waiting a good choice for me?
- Are new treatments under study? Would a clinical trial be appropriate for me?
- What are the expected benefits of each kind of treatment?
- What are the risks and possible side effects of each treatment? How can the side effects be managed?
- Is treatment likely to affect my sex life?
- Am I likely to have urinary problems?
- Am I likely to have bowel problems, such as diarrhea or rectal bleeding?
- Will I need to change my normal activities? If so, for how long?

Methods of Treatment

Treatment for prostate cancer may involve watchful waiting, surgery, radiation therapy, or hormonal therapy. Some patients receive a combination of therapies. In addition, doctors are studying other methods of treatment to find out whether they are effective against this disease.

Watchful waiting may be suggested for some men who have prostate cancer that is found at an early stage and appears to be slow growing. Also, watchful waiting may be advised for older men or men with other serious medical problems. For these men, the risks and possible side effects of surgery, radiation therapy, or hormonal therapy may outweigh the possible benefits. Men with early stage prostate cancer are taking part in a study to determine when or whether treatment may be necessary and effective.

Surgery is a common treatment for early stage prostate cancer. The doctor may remove all of the prostate (a type of surgery called radical prostatectomy) or only part of it. In some cases, the doctor can use a new technique known as nerve-sparing surgery. This type of surgery may save the nerves that control erection. However, men with large tumors or tumors that are very close to the nerves may not be able to have this surgery.

The doctor can describe the types of surgery and can discuss and compare their benefits and risks.

- In *radical retropubic prostatectomy*, the doctor removes the entire prostate and nearby lymph nodes through an incision in the abdomen.

- In *radical perineal prostatectomy*, the doctor removes the entire prostate through an incision between the scrotum and the anus. Nearby lymph nodes are sometimes removed through a separate incision in the abdomen.

- In *transurethral resection of the prostate (TURP)*, the doctor removes part of the prostate with an instrument that is inserted through the urethra. The cancer is cut from the prostate by electricity passing through a small wire loop on the end of the instrument. This method is used mainly to remove tissue that blocks urine flow.

If the pathologist finds cancer cells in the lymph nodes, it is likely that the disease has spread to other parts of the body. Sometimes, the doctor removes the lymph nodes before doing a prostatectomy. If the prostate cancer has not spread to the lymph nodes, the doctor then removes the prostate. But if cancer has spread to the nodes, the doctor usually does not remove the prostate, but may suggest other treatment.

These are some questions a patient may want to ask the doctor before having surgery:

- What kind of operation will I have?

- How will I feel after the operation?

- If I have pain, how will you help?

- How long will I be in the hospital?
- When can I get back to my normal activities?
- Will I have any lasting side effects?
- What is my chance of a full recovery?

Radiation therapy (also called radiotherapy) uses high-energy x-rays to kill cancer cells. Like surgery, radiation therapy is local therapy; it can affect cancer cells only in the treated area. In early stage prostate cancer, radiation can be used instead of surgery, or it may be used after surgery to destroy any cancer cells that may remain in the area. In advanced stages, it may be given to relieve pain or other problems.

Radiation may be directed at the body by a machine (external radiation), or it may come from tiny radioactive seeds placed inside or near the tumor (internal or implant radiation, or brachytherapy). Men who receive radioactive seeds alone usually have small tumors. Some men with prostate cancer receive both kinds of radiation therapy.

For external radiation therapy, patients go to the hospital or clinic, usually 5 days a week for several weeks. Patients may stay in the hospital for a short time for implant radiation.

Hormonal therapy keeps cancer cells from getting the male hormones they need to grow. It is called systemic therapy because it can affect cancer cells throughout the body. Systemic therapy is used to treat cancer that has spread. Sometimes this type of therapy is used to try to prevent the cancer from coming back after surgery or radiation treatment.

There are several forms of hormonal therapy:

- Orchiectomy is surgery to remove the testicles, which are the main source of male hormones.

- Drugs known as a luteinizing hormone-releasing hormone (LH-RH) agonists can prevent the testicles from producing testosterone. Examples are leuprolide, goserelin, and buserelin.

- Drugs known as antiandrogens can block the action of androgens. Two examples are flutamide and bicalutamide.

- Drugs that can prevent the adrenal glands from making androgens include ketoconazole and aminoglutethimide.

After orchiectomy or treatment with an LH-RH agonist, the body no longer gets testosterone from the testicles. However, the adrenal glands still produce small amounts of male hormones. Sometimes, the patient is also given an antiandrogen, which blocks the effect of any remaining male hormones. This combination of treatments is known as total androgen blockade. Doctors do not know for sure whether total androgen blockade is more effective than orchiectomy or LH-RH agonist alone.

Prostate cancer that has spread to other parts of the body usually can be controlled with hormonal therapy for a period of time, often several years. Eventually, however, most prostate cancers are able to grow with very little or no male hormones. When this happens, hormonal therapy is no longer effective, and the doctor may suggest other forms of treatment that are under study.

Side Effects of Treatment

It is hard to limit the effects of treatment so that only cancer cells are removed or destroyed. Because healthy cells and tissues may be damaged, treatment often causes unwanted side effects. Doctors and nurses will explain the possible side effects of treatment.

The side effects of cancer treatment depend mainly on the type and extent of the treatment. Also, each patient reacts differently.

Watchful Waiting

Although men who choose watchful waiting avoid the side effects of surgery and radiation, there can be some negative aspects to this choice. Watchful waiting may reduce the chance of controlling the disease before it spreads. Also, older men should keep in mind that it may be harder to manage surgery and radiation therapy as they age.

Some men may decide against watchful waiting because they feel they would be uncomfortable living with an untreated cancer, even one that appears to be growing slowly or not at all. A man who chooses watchful waiting but later becomes concerned or anxious should discuss his feelings with his doctor. A different treatment approach is nearly always available.

Surgery

Patients are often uncomfortable for the first few days after surgery. Their pain usually can be controlled with medicine, and patients should discuss pain relief with the doctor or nurse. The patient will wear a catheter (a tube inserted into the urethra) to drain urine for 10 days to 3 weeks. The nurse or doctor will show the man how to care for the catheter.

It is also common for patients to feel extremely tired or weak for a while. The length of time it takes to recover from an operation varies. Surgery to remove the prostate may cause long-term problems, including rectal injury or urinary incontinence. Some men may have permanent impotence. Nerve-sparing surgery is an attempt to avoid the problem of impotence. When the doctor can use nerve-sparing surgery and the operation is fully successful, impotence may be only temporary. Still, some men who have this procedure may be permanently impotent.

Men who have a prostatectomy no longer produce semen, so they have dry orgasms. Men who wish to father children may consider sperm banking or a sperm retrieval procedure.

Radiation Therapy

Radiation therapy may cause patients to become extremely tired, especially in the later weeks of treatment. Resting is important, but doctors usually encourage men to try to stay as active as they can. Some men may have diarrhea or frequent and uncomfortable urination.

When men with prostate cancer receive external radiation therapy, it is common for the skin in the treated area to become red, dry, and tender. External radiation therapy can also cause hair loss in the treated area. The loss may be temporary or permanent, depending on the dose of radiation.

Both types of radiation therapy may cause impotence in some men, but internal radiation therapy is not as likely as external radiation therapy to damage the nerves that control erection. However, internal radiation therapy may cause temporary incontinence. Long-term side effects from internal radiation therapy are uncommon.

Hormonal Therapy

The side effects of hormonal therapy depend largely on the type of treatment. Orchiectomy and LH-RH agonists often cause side effects such as impotence, hot flashes, and loss of sexual desire. When first taken, an LH-RH agonist may make a patient's symptoms worse for a short time. This temporary problem is called "flare." Gradually, however, the treatment causes a man's testosterone level to fall. Without testosterone, tumor growth slows down and the patient's condition improves. (To prevent flare, the doctor may give the man an antiandrogen for a while along with the LH-RH agonist.)

Antiandrogens can cause nausea, vomiting, diarrhea, or breast growth or tenderness. If used a long time, ketoconazole may cause liver problems, and aminoglutethimide can cause skin rashes. Men who receive total androgen blockade may experience more side effects than men who receive a single method of hormonal therapy. Any method of hormonal therapy that lowers androgen levels can contribute to weakening of the bones in older men.

Followup Care

During and after treatment, the doctor will continue to follow the patient. The doctor will examine the man regularly to be sure that the disease has not returned or progressed, and will decide what other medical care may be needed. Followup exams may include x-rays, scans, and lab tests, such as the PSA blood test.

Support for Men with Prostate Cancer

Living with a serious disease such as cancer is not easy. Some people find they need help coping with the emotional as well as the practical aspects of their disease. Patients often get together in support groups, where they can share what they have learned about coping with their disease and the effects of treatment. Patients may want to talk with a member of their health care team about finding a support group.

People living with cancer may worry about caring for their families, keeping their jobs, or continuing daily activities. Concerns about treatments and managing side effects, hospital stays, and medical bills are also common. Doctors, nurses, dietitians and other members of the health care team can answer questions about treatment, working, or other activities. Meeting with a social worker, counselor, or member of the clergy can be helpful to those who want to talk about their feelings or discuss their concerns. Often, a social worker can suggest resources for help with rehabilitation, emotional support, financial aid, transportation, or home care.

It is natural for a man and his partner to be concerned about the effects of prostate cancer and its treatment on their sexual relationship. They may want to talk with the doctor about possible side effects and whether these are likely to be temporary or permanent. Whatever the outlook, it is usually helpful for patients and their partners to talk about their concerns and help one another find ways to be intimate during and after treatment.

The Promise of Prostate Cancer Research

Doctors all over the country are conducting many types of clinical trials (research studies) in which people take part voluntarily. These include studies of ways to prevent, detect, diagnose, and treat prostate cancer; studies of the psychological effects of the disease; and studies of ways to improve comfort and quality of life. Research already has led to advances in these areas, and researchers continue to search for more effective approaches.

People who take part in clinical trials have the first chance to benefit from new approaches. They also make important contributions to medical science. Although clinical trials may pose some risks, researchers take very careful steps to protect people who take part.

Causes

Although researchers know several risk factors for prostate cancer, they still are not sure why one man develops the disease and another doesn't.

Some aspects of a man's lifestyle may affect his chances of developing prostate cancer. For example, some evidence suggests a link between diet and this disease. These studies show that prostate cancer is more common in populations that consume a high-fat diet (particularly animal fat), and in populations that have diets lacking certain nutrients. Although it is not known whether a diet low in fat will prevent prostate cancer, a low-fat diet may have many other health benefits.

Some research suggests that high levels of testosterone may increase a man's risk of prostate cancer. The difference between racial groups in prostate cancer risk could be related to high testosterone levels, but it also could result from diet or other lifestyle factors.

Researchers also are looking for changes in genes that may increase the risk for developing prostate cancer. They are studying the genes of men who were diagnosed with prostate cancer at a relatively young age (less than 55 years old) and the genes of families who have several members with the disease. Much more work is needed, however, before scientists can say exactly how changes in these genes are related to prostate cancer. Men with a family history of prostate cancer who are concerned about an inherited risk for this disease should talk with their doctor. The doctor may suggest seeing a health professional trained in genetics.

Prevention

Several studies are under way to explore how prostate cancer might be prevented. These include the use of dietary supplements, such as vitamin E and selenium. In addition, recent studies suggest that a diet that regularly includes tomato-based foods may help protect men from prostate cancer.

The drug finasteride is being studied in the Prostate Cancer Prevention Trial, which involves thousands of men across the country who are participating for 7 years, until 2004.

Scientists are also looking at ways to prevent recurrence among men who have been treated for prostate cancer. These approaches involve the use of drugs such as finasteride, flutamide, and LH-RH agonists. Studies have shown that hormonal therapy after radiation therapy or after radical prostatectomy can benefit certain men whose cancer has spread to nearby tissues.

Researchers also are investigating whether diets that are low in fat and high in soy, fruits, vegetables, and other food products might prevent a recurrence. The Cancer Information Service can provide information about these studies.

Screening/Early Detection

Researchers are studying ways to screen men for prostate cancer (check for the disease in men who have no symptoms). At this time, it is not known whether screening for prostate cancer actually saves lives, even if the disease is found at an earlier stage. The NCI-supported Prostate, Lung, Colorectal, and Ovarian Cancer Screening Trial is designed to show whether certain detection tests can reduce the number of deaths from these cancers. This trial is looking at the usefulness of prostate cancer screening by performing a digital rectal exam and checking the PSA level in the blood in men ages 55 to 74. The results of this trial may change the way men are screened for prostate cancer. The Cancer Information Service can provide information about this trial.

Treatment

Through research, doctors try to find new, more effective ways to treat prostate cancer. Many studies of new approaches for men with prostate cancer are under way. When laboratory research shows that a new treatment method has promise, cancer patients receive the new approach in treatment clinical trials. These studies are designed to answer important questions and to find out whether the new approach is safe and effective. Often, clinical trials compare a new treatment with a standard approach.

Cryosurgery is under study as an alternative to surgery and radiation therapy. The doctor tries to avoid damaging healthy tissue by placing an instrument known as a cryoprobe in direct contact with the tumor to freeze it. The extreme cold destroys the cancer cells.

Doctors are studying new ways of using radiation therapy and hormonal therapy. They also are testing the effectiveness of chemotherapy and biological therapy for men whose cancer does not respond or stops responding to hormonal therapy. In addition, scientists are exploring new treatment schedules and new ways of combining various types of treatment. For example, they are studying the usefulness of hormonal therapy before primary therapy (surgery or radiation) to shrink the tumor.

For men with early stage prostate cancer, researchers also are comparing treatment with watchful waiting. The results of this work will help doctors know whether to treat early stage prostate cancer immediately or only later on, if symptoms occur or worsen.

Chapter 6

Screening for Prostate Cancer

What Is Screening?

Screening for cancer is examination (or testing) of people for early stages in the development of cancer even though they have no symptoms. Scientists have studied patterns of cancer in the population to learn which people are more likely to get certain types of cancer. They have also studied what things around us and what things we do in our lives may cause cancer. This information sometimes helps doctors recommend who should be screened for certain types of cancer, what types of screening tests people should have, and how often these tests should be done. Not all screening tests are helpful, and they often have risks. For this reason, scientists at the National Cancer Institute are studying many screening tests to find out how useful they are and to determine the relative benefits and harms.

If your doctor suggests certain cancer screening tests as part of your health care plan, this does not mean he or she thinks you have cancer. Screening tests are done when you have no symptoms. Since decisions about screening can be difficult, you may want to discuss them with your doctor and ask questions about the potential benefits and risks of screening tests and whether they have been proven to decrease the risk of dying from cancer.

CancerNet, National Cancer Institute (NCI), November 2000.

If your doctor suspects that you may have cancer, he or she will order certain tests to see whether you do. These are called diagnostic tests. Some tests are used for diagnostic purposes, but are not suitable for screening people who have no symptoms.

The purposes of this chapter on prostate cancer screening is to:

- give information on prostate cancer and what makes it more likely to occur (risk factors)

- describe prostate cancer screening methods and what is known about their effectiveness

You can talk to your doctor or health care professional about cancer screening and whether it would be likely to help you.

Screening Tests for Prostate Cancer

- **Digital Rectal Examination**—A digital rectal examination (DRE) is performed by a doctor during a regular office visit. For this examination, the doctor inserts a gloved finger into the rectum and feels the prostate gland through the rectal wall to check for bumps or abnormal areas. Although this test has been used for many years, whether DRE is effective in decreasing the number of deaths from prostate cancer has not been determined.

- **Transrectal Ultrasonography**—During this examination, high-frequency sound waves are sent out by a probe about the size of the index finger, which is inserted into the rectum. The waves bounce off the prostate gland and produce echoes that a computer uses to create a picture called a sonogram. Doctors examine the sonogram for echoes that might represent abnormal areas. Whether ultrasonography is effective in decreasing mortality from prostate cancer has not been determined.

- **PSA**—For this test, a blood sample is drawn and the amount of prostate-specific antigen (PSA) present is determined in a laboratory. PSA is a marker that, if present in higher than average amounts, may indicate prostate cancer cells. However, PSA levels may also be higher in men who have noncancerous prostate conditions. Scientists are studying ways to improve the reliability of the PSA test.

Because unnecessary treatment due to false screening results could be harmful, research is being done to determine the most reliable method for prostate cancer screening. For example, scientists at the National Cancer Institute are studying the value of early detection by DRE and PSA on reducing the number of deaths caused by prostate cancer.

Chapter 7

The Prostate-Specific Antigen (PSA) Test

What is the prostate-specific antigen (PSA) test?

The prostate-specific antigen (PSA) test measures the level of PSA in the blood. A blood sample is drawn and the amount of PSA is measured in a laboratory. PSA is a protein produced by the cells of the prostate gland. When the prostate gland enlarges, PSA levels in the blood tend to rise. PSA levels can rise due to cancer or benign (not cancerous) conditions. Because PSA is produced by the body and can be used to detect disease, it is sometimes called a biological marker or tumor marker.

As men age, both benign prostate conditions and prostate cancer become more frequent. The most common benign prostate conditions are prostatitis (inflammation of the prostate) and benign prostatic hyperplasia (BPH) (enlargement of the prostate). There is no evidence that prostatitis or BPH cause cancer, but it is possible for a man to have one or both of these conditions and to develop prostate cancer as well.

Although PSA levels alone do not give doctors enough information to distinguish between benign prostate conditions and cancer, the doctor will take the result of this test into account in deciding whether to check further for signs of prostate cancer.

Why is the PSA test performed?

The U.S. Food and Drug Administration (FDA) has approved the PSA test for use in conjunction with a digital rectal exam (DRE) to

CancerNet, National Cancer Institute (NCI), 2000.

71

help detect prostate cancer in men age 50 and older. During a DRE, a doctor inserts a gloved finger into the rectum and feels the prostate gland through the rectal wall to check for bumps or abnormal areas. Doctors often use the PSA test and DRE as prostate cancer screening tests in men who have no symptoms of the disease. The FDA has also approved the PSA test to monitor patients with a history of prostate cancer to see if the cancer has come back (recurred).

For whom might a PSA screening test be recommended? How often is testing done?

The benefits of screening for prostate cancer are still being studied. The National Cancer Institute (NCI) is currently conducting the Prostate, Lung, Colorectal, and Ovarian Cancer Screening Trial, or PLCO trial, to determine if certain screening tests reduce the number of deaths from these cancers. The DRE and PSA are being studied to determine whether yearly screening to detect prostate cancer will decrease one's chance of dying from prostate cancer.

Doctors' recommendations for screening vary. Some encourage yearly screening for men over age 50; others recommend against routine screening; still others counsel men about the risks and benefits on an individual basis and encourage patients to make personal decisions about screening. Several risk factors increase a man's chances of developing prostate cancer. These factors may be taken into consideration when a doctor recommends screening. Age is the most common risk factor, with more than 96 percent of prostate cancer cases occurring in men age 55 and older. Other risk factors for prostate cancer include family history and race. Men who have a father or brother with prostate cancer have a greater chance of developing prostate cancer. African American men have the highest rate of prostate cancer, while Native American men have the lowest.

How are PSA test results reported?

PSA test results report the level of PSA detected in the blood. The PSA level that is considered normal for an average man ranges from 0 to 4 nanograms per milliliter (ng/ml). A PSA level of 4 to 10 ng/ml is considered slightly elevated; levels between 10 and 20 ng/ml are considered moderately elevated; and anything above that is considered highly elevated. various factors can cause PSA levels to fluctuate, one abnormal PSA test does not necessarily indicate a need for other diagnostic tests. When PSA levels continue to rise over time, other tests may be indicated.

What if the test results show an elevated PSA level?

A man should discuss elevated PSA test results with his doctor. There are many possible reasons for an elevated PSA level, including prostate cancer, benign prostate enlargement, inflammation, infection, age, and race. If there are no other indicators that suggest cancer, the doctor may recommend repeating DRE and PSA tests regularly to monitor any changes.

If a man's PSA levels have been increasing or if a suspicious lump is detected in the DRE, the doctor may recommend other diagnostic tests to determine if there is cancer or another problem in the prostate. A urine test may be used to detect a urinary tract infection or blood in the urine. The doctor may recommend imaging tests, such as ultrasound (a test in which high-frequency sound waves are used to obtain images of the kidneys and bladder), x-rays, or cystoscopy (a procedure in which a doctor looks into the urethra and bladder through a thin, lighted tube). Medicine or surgery may be recommended if the problem is BPH or an infection.

If cancer is suspected, the only way to tell for sure is to perform a biopsy. For a biopsy, samples of prostate tissue are removed and viewed under a microscope to determine if cancer cells are present. The doctor may use ultrasound to view the prostate during the biopsy, but ultrasound cannot be used alone to tell if cancer is present.

What are some of the limitations of the PSA test?

Detection does not always mean saving lives: Even though the PSA test can detect small tumors, finding a small tumor does not necessarily reduce a man's chance of dying from prostate cancer. PSA testing may identify very slow-growing tumors that are unlikely to threaten a man's life. Also, PSA testing may not help a man with a fast-growing or aggressive cancer that has already spread to other parts of his body before being detected.

False positive tests: False positive test results (also called false positives) occur when the PSA level is elevated, but no cancer is actually present. False positives may lead to additional medical procedures, with significant financial costs and anxiety for the patient and his family. Most men with an elevated PSA test turn out not to have cancer.

False positives occur primarily in men age 50 or older. In this age group, 15 of every 100 men will have elevated PSA levels (higher than 4 ng/ml). Of these 15 men, 12 will be false positives and only three will turn out to have cancer.

False negative tests: False negative test results (also called false negatives) occur when the PSA level is in the normal range even though prostate cancer is actually present. Most prostate cancers are slow-growing and may exist for decades before they are large enough to cause symptoms. Subsequent PSA tests may indicate a problem before the disease progresses significantly.

Why is the PSA test controversial?

Using the PSA test to screen men for prostate cancer is controversial because it is not yet known if the process actually saves lives. Moreover, it is not clear if the benefits of PSA screening outweigh the risks of followup diagnostic tests and cancer treatments.

The procedures used to diagnose prostate cancer may cause significant side effects, including bleeding and infection. Prostate cancer treatment often causes incontinence and impotence. For these reasons, it is important that the benefits and risks of diagnostic procedures and treatment be taken into account when considering whether to undertake prostate cancer screening.

What research is being done to improve the PSA test?

Scientists are researching ways to distinguish between cancerous and benign conditions, and between slow-growing cancers and fast-growing, potentially lethal cancers. Some of the methods being studied are:

- *PSA velocity:* PSA velocity is based on changes in PSA levels over time. A sharp rise in the PSA level raises the suspicion of cancer.

- *Age-adjusted PSA:* Age is an important factor in increasing PSA levels. For this reason, some doctors use age-adjusted PSA levels to determine when diagnostic tests are needed. When age-adjusted PSA levels are used, a different PSA level is defined as normal for each 10-year age group. Doctors who use this method suggest that men younger than age 50 should have a PSA level below 2.5 ng/ml, while a PSA level up to 6.5 ng/ml would be considered normal for men in their 70s. Doctors do not agree about the accuracy and usefulness of age-adjusted PSA levels.

- *PSA density:* PSA density considers the relationship of the PSA level to the size and weight of the prostate. In other words, an elevated PSA might not arouse suspicion in a man with a very enlarged prostate. The use of PSA density to interpret PSA results is controversial because cancer might be overlooked in a man with an enlarged prostate.

- *Free versus attached PSA:* PSA circulates in the blood in two forms: free or attached to a protein molecule. With benign prostate conditions, there is more free PSA, while cancer produces more of the attached form. Researchers are exploring different ways to measure PSA and to compare these measurements to determine if cancer is present.

- *Other screening tests:* Scientists are also developing screening tests for other biological markers, which are not yet commercially available. These markers may be present in higher levels in the blood of men with prostate cancer.

Chapter 8

Questions and Answers about Early Prostate Cancer

This chapter contains a series of questions and answers specific to the early stages of prostate cancer, and will be informative to those seeking information regarding this aspect of the disease.

What is the prostate?

The prostate is a male sex gland, part of a man's reproductive system. The prostate is about the size of a walnut. It is located below the bladder and in front of the rectum.

What is prostate cancer?

Except for skin cancer, cancer of the prostate is the most common malignancy in American men. It is estimated that in 1999 in the United States nearly 179,300 men will be diagnosed with prostate cancer. In the majority of men with prostate cancer, it is very slow growing, and many, if not most, of these men will not die because of the prostate cancer, but rather will live with it until they eventually die of some other cause. Early prostate cancer is localized (confined) to the gland, and the majority of patients with localized prostate cancer have a long survival after diagnosis.

Who is at risk for prostate cancer?

All men are at risk. The most common risk factor is age. More than 75 percent of men diagnosed with prostate cancer each year are over

CancerNet, National Cancer Institute (NCI), 1999.

the age of 65. African American men have a higher risk of prostate cancer than white Americans. Dramatic differences in the incidence of prostate cancer are seen in different countries, and there is some evidence that a diet higher in animal fat may, in part, underlie these differences in risk. Genetic factors also appear to play a role, particularly for families in whom the diagnosis is made in men under 60 years of age. The risk of prostate cancer rises with the number of close relatives who have the disease.

What are the symptoms of prostate cancer?

Prostate cancer often does not cause symptoms for many years. By the time symptoms occur, the disease may have spread beyond the prostate.

When symptoms do occur, they may include:

- Frequent urination, especially at night

- Inability to urinate

- Trouble starting or holding back urination

- A weak or interrupted flow of urine

- Painful or burning urination

- Blood in the urine or semen (the fluid that is released through the penis during orgasm and made up of sperm from the testicles and fluid from the prostate and other sex glands)

- Painful ejaculation (the release of semen through the penis during orgasm)

- Frequent pain or stiffness in the lower back, hips, or upper thighs

These can be symptoms of cancer, but more often they are symptoms of non-cancerous enlargement of the prostate. It is important to check with a doctor.

What other prostate conditions can cause symptoms like these?

The above symptoms may be caused by a variety of conditions. As men get older, their prostate may grow bigger and block the flow of urine or interfere with sexual function. This common condition, called benign prostatic hyperplasia (BPH), is not cancer, but can cause many of the same symptoms as prostate cancer. Although BPH may not be a threat to life, it may require treatment with medicine or surgery to relieve symptoms. Again, it is important to check with a doctor.

Can prostate cancer be found before a man has symptoms?

Yes. Two tests are commonly used to detect prostate cancer in the absence of any symptoms. One is the digital rectal exam, in which a doctor feels the prostate through the rectum to find hard or lumpy areas. The other is a blood test used to detect a substance made by the prostate called prostate specific antigen (PSA). Together, these tests can detect many silent prostate cancers, those that have not caused symptoms.

Currently, the National Cancer Institute is supporting research to learn more about screening men for prostate cancer. This research will try to determine whether the blood test for PSA along with digital rectal examination can help reduce the death rate from this disease. It will also assess the risks and benefits of screening. At present, it is unclear whether routine screening of men who are not at unusually high risk will prove to save lives and outweigh the extra surgery, radiation, and complications of therapy for large numbers of patients, many of whom do not have aggressive or life-threatening tumors.

How reliable are the two tests?

Neither of the screening tests for prostate cancer is perfect. Most men with mildly elevated PSA do not have prostate cancer, and many men with prostate cancer have normal levels of PSA. Also, the digital rectal exam can miss many prostate cancers.

How is prostate cancer diagnosed?

The diagnosis of prostate cancer can be confirmed only by a microscopic examination to identify cancerous prostate tissue. This is done by a biopsy performed in the doctor's office. Prostate cancer is characterized by both grade and stage. Grade is a term used to describe how closely a tumor resembles normal tissue. Based on the microscopic appearance of a tumor, pathologists (doctors who identify diseases by studying tissues under a microscope) may describe it as low-, medium-, or high-grade cancer. One way of grading prostate cancer, called the Gleason system, uses scores of 2 to 10. Another system uses G1 through G4. The higher the score, the higher the grade of the tumor. High-grade tumors grow more quickly and are more likely to spread than low-grade tumors. Staging of prostate cancer means determining the site and location of the disease. Early prostate cancer, stages 1 and 2, is localized to the prostate gland. Stage 3 prostate cancer is locally advanced outside the gland. Stage 4 prostate cancer has spread to other organs or tissues.

How is localized prostate cancer treated?

There are three generally accepted options for treatment of patients with localized prostate cancer: radical prostatectomy, radiation therapy, and surveillance (also called watchful waiting).Radical prostatectomy is a surgical procedure to remove the entire prostate gland and nearby tissues. Sometimes lymph nodes in the pelvic area (the lower part of the abdomen, located between the hip bones) are also removed. Radical prostatectomy may be performed using a technique called nerve-sparing surgery that may prevent damage to the nerves needed for an erection and prevent damage to the opening of the bladder.

Radiation therapy involves the delivery of radiation energy to the prostate. The energy is usually delivered in an outpatient setting using an external beam of radiation. The energy can also be delivered by placing radioactive seeds in the prostate during a surgical procedure.

A third option, surveillance, is recommended by doctors for some patients, particularly those who are older or have other medical conditions that are likely to compromise their health. These patients are followed with regular examinations. If there is evidence of cancer growth, active treatment may be recommended.

How does a patient decide what is the best treatment option for localized prostate cancer?

Choosing a treatment option involves the patient and his family and doctor. Considerations include the grade and stage of the cancer, the patient's age and health, and the individual choices that each patient makes about the benefits and risks of each treatment option. Because there are several reasonable treatment options for most patients, the decision can be difficult. Patients may hear different opinions and recommendations. They should try to get as much information as possible. There is rarely a need to make a decision without time to understand the pros and cons of various approaches.

Chapter 9

What Women Should Know about the Prostate

Introduction

A newborn male has a 13 percent chance of developing prostate cancer during his lifetime and a 3 percent chance of dying of it. These numbers are very similar to the numbers in breast cancer. A new diagnosis of prostate cancer is made in the United States every three minutes and a man dies of it every 15 minutes. Prostate cancer is the only cancer in which death rates are continuing to increase and that's because men are living longer. Men used to die at age 72 of a heart attack, and they now have an angioplasty and die several years later of prostate cancer.

There are three very important diseases of the prostate. Most men don't even know they have a prostate until they develop one of them because the prostate does not have an important physiologic function. Where is the prostate and what does it do? It is a walnut-sized gland, located at the base of the bladder. What is its function? You know the breast is a gland of reproduction and the prostate is also a gland of reproduction. In the reproductive function in men, the prostate provides some of the fluid for the semen. The major function of this fluid may be to prevent urinary tract infections in men.

Why is the prostate important? It is important because it is the source of three of the most important diseases that men develop:

---

prostate cancer, the most common cancer in men; benign enlargement (BPH), the most common benign tumor in men, which produces urinary symptoms in 75 percent of men older than the age of 50; and prostatitis, the most common cause of urinary tract infection in men.

Prostate cancer can be, and usually is, diagnosed at an early, curable stage and treated with fewer side effects than in the past. Furthermore, research promises to provide new ways in the future to prevent the disease, to diagnose it earlier, and to treat it more effectively when advanced.

Benign enlargement can now be treated more safely and less invasively with medicine and surgery, and these approaches are certain to improve in the future. And finally, modern antibiotics are very effective in treating bacterial prostatitis, but new approaches are necessary to understand the cause of nonbacterial disease before effective treatments can be developed.

Does benign enlargement (BPH) progress to cancer?

No. The two diseases arise in different portions of the prostate. A man with BPH is no more, but no less, likely to get cancer, and the reverse is true also.

Should PSA testing be done before age 40?

I don't think so. However, if I were in a family that had a very strong family history, three or more affected members, and I was in my 30s, I probably would get my PSA checked. But there's no strong recommendation that this should be done.

How do you determine what the top age level is to operate for cancer?

Age is a very important factor. First, it is the single best predictor of how long you're going to live. Second, older men, older than the age of 70, have more complications after surgery, such as incontinence. Many men don't appreciate this. They want to live forever. Then they have an operation and they're incontinent, and say, "Why did I do that?" And third, older men often times have more advanced disease. It's been there longer. So patients older than the age of 70 are not ideal candidates for surgery, because they are less likely to live long enough to need to be cured, they may have more advanced disease, and they may have more side effects from surgery. So, I believe that patients in their 70s ideally should be treated with external beam radiotherapy.

The flip side of it is the young, healthy man in his 40s and 50s who should be treated with surgery. And then there are patients in their 60s, where the vast majority of men are, and they have an option. Some men want to get rid of this cancer, and there's no better way than to have it removed. And there are other men who don't want to have an operation. That's where the individual becomes the deciding force in what to do.

Do you use the chronological age of 70?

That's a good point. There's no question that we need a better co-morbidity index. If you have diabetes, have hypertension, smoke cigarettes, have a high-fat diet, don't exercise, and have more than four drinks of alcohol a day, you're not going to live long enough to die of prostate cancer, even if you are 60. On the other hand, if you exercise regularly, have a low-fat, high-fiber diet, and have a high HDL, you may be one of the 70-year-old men who will live to be 100. I'll do a radical prostatectomy on any 80-year-old-man who is brought into the office by both of his parents.

My husband's PSA is high but his biopsy was negative. They told him just to be followed up. Is that OK?

Yes. Let's go through this scenario, because this is the common one. What if the biopsy is negative. What do you do next? Can we say he doesn't have cancer? No. We just took six little cores, or eight little cores at the most. We did not sample the entire prostate. But if one is followed up at six monthly intervals, that is usually sufficient. The PSA should not go up more then 1.5 over a two-year period. That's 0.75 a year, and that's based on some very nice studies done at the Baltimore Longitudinal Study of Aging here at Johns Hopkins by Dr. Ballentine Carter. If it accelerates more than that, then that's an early warning that there is something growing faster than benign disease and it wasn't sampled, and he needs another biopsy.

Does sunlight prevent prostate cancer?

What about sunlight? What did I say? I said that there is an association between a high death rate of prostate cancer in the areas where the sun doesn't shine very much, and a low death rate where it does. Should we all move to California? No.

The problem with associations is that they are just that. We do not know that they are causative. The reason I showed you that data is that prostate cancer is an example of some very interesting epidemiological data, which may some day give insight into what causes it, and most importantly, what could prevent it.

At autopsy, half of the men in the United States have a little prostate cancer. And guess what? In Japan half of the men at autopsy have a little bit of prostate cancer. Men who live in Japan have a low rate of developing prostate cancer, but when they move to the United States it increases, so the initial phase, whatever turns it on, is present in men universally around the world. The first step in developing cancer is initiation; the next one is promotion, what makes it grow. In Japan there's something in their diet or their environment, that prevents prostate cancer from growing. It's either something they don't eat—fat—or something they do eat—green tea—or something else that we don't understand.

I heard somewhere that a son of a woman who had breast cancer may have a higher risk of prostate cancer.

There are two genes, the BRCA1 and the BRCA2, that cause breast cancer. And when researchers evaluated these families, they've found a slightly higher frequency of prostate cancer in the males in those families. We have looked now at a large number of men with hereditary prostate cancer, and found no increased breast cancer in their mothers or sisters. So there may be a very low frequency, but I don't think it's high enough to alert men that they are at the highest risk.

How do you treat nonbacterial prostatitis?

The first thing you do is get the patient's confidence. Rule out all of the other things that might be going through his mind, like cancer and infection. Then you sit down and you talk heart to heart. I'll tell the patient that I'm going to try to treat him symptomatically. Young men don't like that. They want to have this thing cured. They want to get rid of it. But there is no way to get rid of it. And very commonly, if you get someone's confidence, you can treat them with anti-inflammatory agents, you can treat them with alpha blockers, you can treat them with sedatives, you can have them take hot baths, you can have them get involved in something else. Over time, that disease eventually goes away; but it is not easy to do.

My husband had a radical prostatectomy and is impotent. He won't let me help him.

Normally, after a radical prostatectomy, the sensation of sexual activity should be normal and the ability to achieve an orgasm should be normal. Your husband is lucky to have a wonderful wife who wants to help him. Tell him the thing to do is to resume your intimate relationship.

If the nerves were cut, how can sensation ever be normal?

The nerves responsible for sensation are not the nerves that are involved in this operation. The sensory nerves are always there (the pudendal nerve). They are out of the way of the surgery and for this reason sensation, orgasm and sex drive should be normal. The nerves that were severed are nerves that carry no sensory fibers.

My husband has a PSA that keeps going up, but his ultrasound is normal. What should be done?

He needs a biopsy. An ultrasound alone is not good enough.

Chapter 10

The Urinary System and How It Works

Your body takes nutrients from food and uses them to maintain all bodily functions including energy and self-repair. After your body has taken what it needs from the food, waste products are left behind in the blood and in the bowel. The urinary system works with the lungs, skin, and intestines—all of which also excrete wastes—to keep the chemicals and water in your body balanced. Adults eliminate about a quart and a half of urine each day. The amount depends on many factors, the major ones being the amount of fluid and foods a person consumes and how much fluid is lost through sweat and breathing. Certain types of medications can also affect the amount of urine eliminated.

The urinary system removes a type of waste called urea from your blood. Urea is produced when foods containing protein, such as meat, poultry, and certain vegetables, are broken down in the body. Urea is carried in the bloodstream to the kidneys.

The kidneys are bean-shaped organs about the size of your fists. They are near the middle of the back, just below the rib cage. The kidneys remove urea from the blood through tiny filtering units called nephrons. Each nephron consists of a ball formed of small blood capillaries, called a glomerulus, and a small tube called a renal tubule. Urea, together with water and other waste substances, forms the urine as it passes through the nephrons and down the renal tubules of the kidney.

National Institute of Health (NIH) Publication No. 98-3195, April 1998.

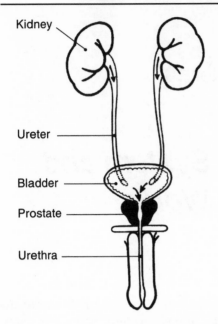

Kidney

Ureter

Bladder

Prostate

Urethra

Figure 10.1. Front View of the Urinary Tract

From the kidneys, urine travels down two thin tubes called ureters to the bladder. The ureters are about 8 to 10 inches long. Muscles in the ureter walls constantly tighten and relax to force urine downward away from the kidneys. If urine is allowed to stand still, or back up, a kidney infection can develop. Small amounts of urine are emptied into the bladder from the ureters about every 10 to 15 seconds.

The bladder is a hollow muscular organ shaped like a balloon. It sits in your pelvis and is held in place by ligaments attached to other organs and the pelvic bones. The bladder stores urine until you are ready to go to the bathroom to empty it. It swells into a round shape when it is full and gets smaller when empty. If the urinary system is healthy, the bladder can hold up to 16 ounces (2 cups) of urine comfortably for 2 to 5 hours.

Circular muscles called sphincters help keep urine from leaking. The sphincter muscles close tightly like a rubber band around the opening of the bladder into the urethra, the tube that allows urine to pass outside the body.

Nerves in the bladder tell you when it is time to urinate (empty your bladder). As the bladder first fills with urine, you may notice a feeling that you need to urinate. The sensation to urinate becomes stronger as the bladder continues to fill and reaches its limit. At that point, nerves from the bladder send a message to the brain that the bladder is full, and your urge to empty your bladder intensifies.

When you urinate, the brain signals the bladder muscles to tighten, squeezing urine out of the bladder. At the same time, the brain signals the sphincter muscles to relax. As these muscles relax, urine exits the bladder through the urethra. When all the signals occur in the correct order, normal urination occurs.

What Causes Problems in the Urinary System?

Problems in the urinary system can be caused by aging, illness, or injury. As you get older, changes in the kidneys' structure cause them to lose some of their ability to remove wastes from the blood. Also, the muscles in your ureters, bladder, and urethra tend to lose some of their strength. You may have more urinary infections because the bladder muscles do not tighten enough to empty your bladder completely. A decrease in strength of muscles of the sphincters and the pelvis can also cause incontinence, the unwanted leakage of urine. Illness or injury can also prevent the kidneys from filtering the blood completely or block the passage of urine.

How Are Problems in the Urinary System Detected?

Urinalysis is a test that studies the content of urine for abnormal substances such as protein or signs of infection. This test involves urinating into a special container and leaving the sample to be studied.

Urodynamic tests evaluate the storage of urine in the bladder and the flow of urine from the bladder through the urethra. Your doctor may want to do a urodynamic test if you are having symptoms that suggest problems with the muscles or nerves of your lower urinary system and pelvis (ureters, bladder, urethra, and sphincter muscles).

Urodynamic tests measure the contraction of the bladder muscle as it fills and empties. The test is done by inserting a small tube called a catheter through your urethra into your bladder to fill it either with water or a gas. Another small tube is inserted into your rectum to measure the pressure put on your bladder when you strain or cough. Other bladder tests use x-ray dye instead of water so that x-ray pictures can be taken when the bladder fills and empties to detect any abnormalities in the shape and function of the bladder. These tests take about an hour.

What Are Some Disorders of the Urinary System?

Disorders of the urinary system range in severity from easy-to-treat to life-threatening. Benign prostatic hyperplasia (BPH) is a condition in men that affects the prostate gland, which is part of the male reproductive system. The prostate is located at the bottom of the bladder and surrounds the urethra. BPH is an enlargement of the prostate gland that can interfere with urinary function in older men. It causes blockage by squeezing the urethra, which can make it difficult to urinate. Men with BPH frequently have other bladder symptoms including an increase in frequency of bladder emptying both during the day and at night. Most men over age 60 have some BPH, but not all have problems with blockage. There are many different treatment options for BPH.

Interstitial cystitis (IC) is a chronic bladder disorder also known as painful bladder syndrome and frequency-urgency-dysuria syndrome. In this disorder, the bladder wall can become inflamed and irritated. The inflammation can lead to scarring and stiffening of the bladder, decreased bladder capacity, pinpoint bleeding, and, in rare cases, ulcers in the bladder lining. The cause of IC is unknown at this time.

Kidney stones is the term commonly used to refer to stones, or calculi, in the urinary system. Stones form in the kidneys and may be found anywhere in the urinary system. They vary in size. Some stones cause great pain while others cause very little. The aim of treatment is to remove the stones, prevent infection, and prevent recurrence. Both nonsurgical and surgical treatments are used. Kidney stones affect men more often than women.

Prostatitis is inflammation of the prostate gland that results in urinary frequency and urgency, burning or painful urination (dysuria), and pain in the lower back and genital area, among other symptoms. In some cases, prostatitis is caused by bacterial infection and can be treated with antibiotics. But the more common forms of prostatitis are not associated with any known infecting organism. Antibiotics are often ineffective in treating the nonbacterial forms of prostatitis.

Proteinuria is the presence of abnormal amounts of protein in the urine. Healthy kidneys take wastes out of the blood but leave in protein. Protein in the urine does not cause a problem by itself. But it may be a sign that your kidneys are not working properly.

Renal (kidney) failure results when the kidneys are not able to regulate water and chemicals in the body or remove waste products from your blood. Acute renal failure (ARF) is the sudden onset of kidney failure. This can be caused by an accident that injures the kidneys, loss of a lot of blood, or some drugs or poisons. ARF may lead to permanent loss of kidney function. But if the kidneys are not seriously damaged, they may recover. Chronic renal failure (CRF) is the gradual reduction of kidney function that may lead to permanent kidney failure, or end-stage renal disease (ESRD). You may go several years without knowing you have CRF.

Urinary tract infections (UTIs) are caused by bacteria in the urinary tract. Women get UTIs more often than men. UTIs are treated with antibiotics. Drinking lots of fluids also helps by flushing out the bacteria.

The name of the UTI depends on its location in the urinary tract. An infection in the bladder is called cystitis. If the infection is in one or both of the kidneys, the infection is called pyelonephritis. This type of UTI can cause serious damage to the kidneys if it is not adequately treated.

Urinary incontinence, loss of bladder control, is the involuntary passage of urine. There are many causes and types of incontinence, and many treatment options. Treatments range from simple exercises to surgery. Women are affected by urinary incontinence more often than men.

Urinary retention, or bladder-emptying problems, is a common urological problem with many possible causes. Normally, urination can be initiated voluntarily and the bladder empties completely. Urinary retention is the abnormal holding of urine in the bladder. Acute urinary retention is the sudden inability to urinate, causing pain and discomfort. Causes can include an obstruction in the urinary system, stress, or neurologic problems. Chronic urinary retention refers to the persistent presence of urine left in the bladder after incomplete emptying. Common causes of chronic urinary retention are bladder muscle failure, nerve damage, or obstructions in the urinary tract. Treatment for urinary retention depends on the cause.

Who Can Help Me With a Urinary Problem?

Your primary doctor can help you with some urinary problems. Your pediatrician may be able to treat some of your child's urinary problems. But some problems may require the attention of a urologist, a doctor who specializes in treating problems of the urinary system and the male reproductive system. A gynecologist is a doctor who specializes in the female reproductive system and may be able to help with some urinary problems. A urogynecologist is a gynecologist who specializes in the female urinary system. A nephrologist specializes in treating diseases of the kidney.

Points To Remember

- Your urinary system filters waste and extra fluid from your blood.

- Problems in the urinary system include kidney failure, urinary tract infections, kidney stones, prostate enlargement, and bladder control problems.

- Health professionals who treat urinary problems include general practitioners (your primary doctor), pediatricians, urologists, gynecologists, urogynecologists, and nephrologists.

Resources for More Information

American Foundation for Urologic Disease
1128 N. Charles Street
Baltimore, MD 21201
Toll Free: 800-242-2383
Tel: 410-468-1800
Fax: 410-468-1808
Internet: http://www.afud.org
E-Mail: admin@afud.org

American Kidney Fund
6110 Executive Boulevard
Suite 1010
Rockville, MD 20852
Toll Free: 800-638-8299
Tel: 301-881-3052
Internet: http://www.akfinc.org
E-Mail: helpline@akfinc.org

American Society of Pediatric Nephrology
Department of Pediatrics
University of Wisconsin Children's Hospital
600 Highland Avenue
Madison, WI 53792-4108
Tel: 608-265-6020
Internet: http://www.aspneph.com

American Uro-Gynecologic Society
401 North Michigan Avenue
Chicago, IL 60611-4267
Tel: 312-644-6610 ext. 4712
Internet: http://www.augs.org
E-Mail: augs@dc.sba.com

Interstitial Cystitis Association
51 Monroe Street
Suite 1402
Rockville, MD 20850
Toll Free: 800-HELP-ICA
Tel: 301-610-5300
Fax: 301-610-5308
Internet: http://www.ichelp.org
E-Mail: icamail@ichelp.org

National Association for Continence (NAFC)
P.O. Box 8310
Spartanburg, SC 29305-8306
Toll Free: 800-BLADDER (800-252-3337)
Tel: 864-579-7900
Fax: 864-579-7902
Internet: http://www.nafc.org
E-Mail: memberservices@nafc.org

National Kidney Foundation
30 East 33rd Street
New York, NY 10016
Toll Free: 800-622-9010
Internet: http://www.kidney.org

The Prostatitis Foundation
Information Distribution Center
Parkway Business Center
2029 Ireland Grove Road
Bloomington, IL 61704
Tel: 309-664-6222
Internet: http://www.prostate.org
E-Mail: Mcapstone@aol.com

The Simon Foundation for Continence
P.O. Box 835
Wilmette, IL 60091
Toll Free: 800-23-SIMON
Tel: 847-864-3913 (main office)
Internet: http://www.simonfoundation.org
E-Mail: simoninfo@simonfoundation.org

Part Three

Treatment of Prostate Cancer

Chapter 11

Understanding Treatment Choices for Prostate Cancer

One of the first questions a patient with prostate cancer will usually ask is "what are my treatment choices?" This answer has become increasingly complex as progress has been made in prostate cancer treatment. A wide variety of therapies are now available, each with its own promises and limitations. This chapter will present you with an overview of modern prostate cancer management.

The major determinant of therapy is whether cancer has spread beyond the prostate or not. If all of the cancer is in the prostate gland, treatment is directed to that organ. If cancer is detected outside the prostate, treatment must reach other parts of the body.

Treatment may be said to be "curative" or "palliative."

- *Curative* therapy is aimed at completely eliminating cancer from the patient's body. If this is successful, the tumor will not recur after treatment, and the patient's life expectancy should be the same as if he never had cancer.

- In *palliative* therapy, the goal is not to cure the cancer. Instead, treatments are intended to slow down progression of the cancer or relieve specific complications. When a cure is not possible, palliative therapy can greatly improve quality of life, and often extend it considerably.

"Prostate Cancer Treatment Options," by David A. Cooke, MD. © 2001 Omnigraphics, Inc.

Managing Cancers Limited to the Prostate Gland

When there does not appear to be any cancer outside of the prostate gland, chances for cure are best. There may be a real possibility of destroying all of the cancer cells, eliminating it from the body. Accordingly, therapies for limited cancers focus on the prostate gland. Sometimes, a combination of treatments can give superior results.

Watchful Waiting

For some men, the best treatment is no treatment at all. It has become increasingly understood that many more men die *with* prostate cancer than *of* prostate cancer. Some men have very slow-growing cancers which do not cause symptoms or spread outside the prostate gland. Such men may live to an advanced age, and finally die from another cause completely unrelated to their cancer. This is a preferred option for very elderly men, or men in poor health, but it may be chosen by younger men as well. It is a gamble, but it is ideal for some patients who have the odds stacked in their favor.

Surgical Therapy

This was the first treatment for prostate cancer, and it remains important today. During an operation, the cancer and the prostate gland are removed. Surgery appears to offer the best chance for a cure of prostate cancer.

There are problems, however. Surgery involves considerable physical stress, and can cause a heart attack, pneumonia, or stroke. Anatomy creates other limitations. The bladder and the nerve supply to the penis both lay very close to the prostate. Some men become impotent or incontinent if they are damaged during surgery.

Several different kinds of prostate cancer surgery are available. These include:

- *Radical Prostatectomy:* Complete removal of the prostate gland and some of the surrounding tissue.

- *Retropubic Prostatectomy:* A different approach which allows the surgeon to inspect and remove lymph nodes in the pelvis in addition to removing the prostate.

- *Perineal Prostatectomy:* Surgery through an incision between the penis and the rectum. It may cause less bleeding than other types.

- *Nerve-Sparing Surgery:* An attempt to preserve the nerves to the penis which pass through the prostate gland. It may cause fewer sexual problems after surgery, but outcomes have been mixed.

- *Cryosurgery, Radiosurgery, and Microwave Surgery:* Techniques which destroy cancer tissue by freezing or burning. These are usually done without an incision through the penis, under sedation. They are new, and it is unclear how they compare to other forms of surgery.

Radiation Therapy

Radiation damages cells, and will kill them if given in sufficient doses. Cancer cells are usually damaged more easily than normal cells, so they can be killed selectively. In some cases, they can be eliminated completely. Radiation therapy is not as likely to cure prostate cancer as surgery, but it can be quite effective.

It also has its drawbacks. Radiation damages the cancer more than healthy tissue, but it does damage healthy tissue. Burns, scarring, and temporary or persistent inflammation may result. Impotence and incontinence can also occur, but much less often than with surgery.

There are two general kinds of radiation therapy: external beam and internal radiation.

- *External Beam:* After careful positioning in a large machine, several precisely-targeted radiation beams are aimed at the cancer for seconds to minutes. The treatment is repeated multiple times over weeks. The goal is to direct maximum radiation to the cancer, and minimal radiation to normal tissue.

- *Internal Radiation:* A newer technique which involves placing small radioactive "seeds" in the prostate. These tiny capsules of radioactive material release radiation directly into the prostate gland, without passing through other structures. It has fewer side effects and results in less damage to healthy tissue than external beam radiation. Internal radiation works best with clearly localized tumors.

Medications

Medication may be used for treatment of prostate cancer, most often in combination with surgery or radiation. It is not generally

99

recommended as first-line treatment in men with localized prostate cancer. The following section will discuss medication in more detail.

Management of Cancers that Have Spread Outside the Gland

Prostate cancer may have spread outside the gland by the time it is discovered. This changes management, since treatment can't be directed just at the prostate. It also reduces the odds of a cure, since it becomes difficult to kill all the cancerous cells. As a result, care is more likely to be palliative in nature.

Medication Therapy

Medication therapy is frequently used in advanced prostate cancer. Because medications travel through the bloodstream to all parts of the body, they can affect tumor cells anywhere. There are two general categories: hormonal therapy and chemotherapy.

Hormonal Therapy

Most prostate cancers sense male hormones in the blood. In fact, some require these hormones to grow. Shutting off the supply of male hormones may dramatically slow cancer growth. This is sometimes referred to as "chemical castration."

Several classes of drugs have been developed that deprive prostate cancer cells of hormone stimulation. Leuprolide and buserelin stop hormone production in the brain. Others, such as aminoglutethimide, stop hormone production elsewhere in the body. Flutamide and cyproteone prevent cancer cells from detecting male hormones in the blood. Estrogen, a female hormone, can also be given to men to slow prostate cancer growth.

These medications can be quite effective, especially when used in combination with surgery or radiation. They rarely produce cures by themselves. Because they interfere with male hormones, they can cause loss of sex drive, impotence and hot flashes.

Chemotherapy

Chemotherapy is an attempt to selectively poison cancer cells. Unfortunately, chemotherapy does not work well for prostate cancer. It is usually reserved for when other options fail. Side effects vary considerably depending on which drugs are used. Commonly, they include anemia, hair loss, nausea, and vomiting.

Surgical Therapy

Surgical orchiectomy (castration) may be recommended. The testicles are removed, but the penis is left intact. The testicles are the major source of male hormones in the body, and when they are removed, hormone levels drop dramatically. This operation has become less common since the advent of anti-hormone medications, but it remains an option for some men.

Radiation Therapy

Radiation therapy can be very helpful in treating advanced prostate cancer. For example, tumor spread into bone may cause pain and can lead to fracture. External beam radiation to an affected bone may dramatically relieve pain and improve ability to function.

"Alternative" or "Complementary" Therapy

In recent years, there has been increased interest in the general public in nontraditional treatments for disease conditions, including cancer. These encompass a wide variety of techniques, including special diets, detoxifying regimens, herbal supplements, vitamins, and homeopathy. They can be very appealing, especially when "mainstream" therapies carry significant risks and side effects.

Unfortunately, none of these therapies have scientific support. Little is known about their safety or efficacy. Some are undoubtedly frauds, victimizing desperate people to take their money. Others may be honest, but worthless. Still others may be genuinely helpful, and will eventually become "mainstream." Without scientific study, it is difficult to tell them apart.

If you are interested in trying an "alternative" or "complementary" therapy, there are a few guidelines to keep in mind. First, always discuss your plans with your doctor. Some "alternative" remedies can interact or interfere with treatments you are receiving with your doctor. Second, understand that any therapy, even if "herbal" or "natural" can hurt you. Third, be very suspicious of "secret formulas" or "breakthrough" treatments, especially when accompanied by large numbers of "testimonials." Often, they will claim to be suppressed by the medical "establishment." These are usually frauds.

Conclusions

Many options exist for men diagnosed with prostate cancer. The following chapters will discuss the details of individual therapies in more detail.

Prostate Cancer Treatment Glossary

In discussing treatment, it is important to understand some of the more commonly-used medical terms. Some pertaining to prostate cancer include:

PSA (Prostate Specific Antigen): A substance detectable in the blood that is normally produced by cells in the prostate gland. Prostate cancer cells often make large amounts of this substance. Blood levels of PSA may be used to diagnose prostate cancer, and are frequently used to monitor response to anti-cancer treatment.

Gleason Score: A number between two and ten assigned by a pathologist who has examined biopsy specimens from a patient with prostate cancer. This score helps predict how aggressive (likely to spread) the tumor will be. Higher numbers indicate a more dangerous cancer.

Tumor Grade: Similar to the Gleason Score above, this is a estimate of how likely a given case of prostate cancer is to spread into other tissues. This is determined by looking at the biopsy sample, and comparing its appearance to tumors from other people. The grade is usually given as a number from zero to four, with four being the worst. Grade says nothing about how far a tumor has already spread; it simply says how likely it is to spread if it is not treated.

Tumor Stage: A measure of how much the tumor has already spread. This is usually determined by X-ray studies. For prostate cancer, this is expressed as letters A through D. Stage A means the cancer is confined to only a small part of the prostate, while Stage D means the cancer has spread to organs in other parts of the body.

5-Year Survival: This is often used to compare different kinds of treatment for prostate cancer. It is the percentage of patients who can expect to still be alive five years after a given treatment. It is not a "cure" rate; it is simply the odds of surviving five years, with or without cancer.

—by David A. Cooke, M.D.

Chapter 12

Cryosurgery

Cryosurgery (also called cryotherapy) is the use of extreme cold to destroy cancer cells. Traditionally, it has been used to treat external tumors, such as those on the skin, but recently some physicians have begun using it as a treatment for tumors that occur inside the body. Cryosurgery for internal tumors is increasing as a result of developments in technology over the past several years.

For external tumors, liquid nitrogen (-196 degrees Celsius, -320.8 degrees Fahrenheit) is applied directly to the cancer cells with a cotton swab or spraying device. For internal tumors, liquid nitrogen is circulated through an instrument called a cryoprobe, which is placed in contact with the tumor. To guide the cryoprobe and to monitor the freezing of the cells, the physician uses ultrasound (computerized moving pictures of the body generated by high-frequency sound waves). By using ultrasound, physicians hope to spare nearby healthy tissue.

Cryosurgery often involves a cycle of treatments in which the tumor is frozen, allowed to thaw, and then refrozen.

Cryosurgery is being evaluated in the treatment of a number of cancers, including prostate cancer and cancer that affects the liver (both primary liver cancer and cancer that has spread to the liver from another site). Researchers also are studying its effectiveness as a treatment for some tumors of the bone, for brain and spinal tumors, and for tumors in the windpipe that may develop with non-small cell lung cancer. In addition, some researchers are using cryosurgery in

CancerNet, National Cancer Institute (NCI), 1997.

combination with other cancer treatments such as radiation, surgery, and hormone therapy. While initial results of cryosurgical treatment are encouraging, researchers have not yet drawn any solid conclusions regarding its long-term effectiveness.

For certain types of cancer and precancerous conditions, however, cryosurgery has proven to be an effective therapy. It has traditionally been used to treat retinoblastoma (a childhood cancer that affects the retina of the eye) and early-stage skin cancers (both basal cell and squamous cell carcinomas). Precancerous skin growths known as actinic keratosis and the precancerous condition cervical intraepithelial neoplasia (abnormal cell changes in the cervix that can develop into cervical cancer) also can be treated with cryosurgery.

Cryosurgery in the Treatment of Prostate Cancer

Cryosurgery may be used to treat men with early-stage cancer that is confined to the prostate gland, particularly when standard treatments such as surgery and radiation are unsuccessful or cannot be used. For men in good physical condition with cancer limited to the prostate, however, the standard treatments of prostatectomy (surgical removal of the prostate) or radiation therapy are usually considered better options. Cryosurgery is not considered an effective treatment for prostate cancer that has spread outside the gland, or to distant parts of the body.

In addition, although cryosurgery may be considered an alternative to surgery or radiation therapy in a limited number of cases, its long-term effectiveness has not been demonstrated conclusively.

Complications and Side Effects

Cryosurgery does have side effects, although they may be less severe than those associated with surgery or radiation therapy. Cryosurgery in the liver may cause damage to the bile ducts and/or major blood vessels, which can lead to hemorrhage (heavy bleeding) or infection.

Cryosurgery for prostate cancer may affect the urinary system. It also may cause incontinence (lack of control over urine flow) and impotence (loss of sexual function), although these side effects are often temporary. Cryosurgery for cervical intraepithelial neoplasia has not been shown to affect fertility, but this possibility is under study. More studies must be conducted to determine the long-term effects of cryosurgery.

Advantages and Disadvantages of Cryosurgery

Cryosurgery offers some advantages over other methods of cancer treatment. It is less invasive than surgery, involving only a small incision or insertion of the cryoprobe through the skin. Consequently, pain, bleeding, and other complications of surgery are minimized. Cryosurgery is less expensive than other treatments and requires shorter recovery time and a shorter hospital stay.

Because physicians can focus cryosurgical treatment on a limited area, they can avoid the destruction of nearby healthy tissue. The treatment can be safely repeated and may be used along with standard treatments such as surgery, chemotherapy, and radiation. Furthermore, cryosurgery may offer an option for treating cancers that are considered inoperable or that do not respond to standard treatments.

The major disadvantage of cryosurgery is the uncertainty surrounding its long-term effectiveness. While cryosurgery may be effective in treating tumors made visible to the physician through imaging tests (tests that produce pictures of areas inside the body), it can miss microscopic cancer spread. Furthermore, because the effectiveness of the technique is still being assessed, insurance coverage issues may arise.

The Future of Cryosurgery

Additional studies are needed to determine the effectiveness of cryosurgery in controlling cancer and improving survival. Data from these studies will allow physicians to compare cryosurgery with standard treatment options such as surgery, chemotherapy, and radiation. Moreover, physicians continue to examine the possibility of using cryosurgery in combination with other treatments.

Cryosurgery is widely available in gynecologists' offices for the treatment of cervical neoplasias. A limited number of hospitals and cancer centers throughout the country currently have skilled physicians and the necessary technology to perform cryosurgery for other precancerous and cancerous conditions. Individuals can consult with their doctors or contact hospitals and cancer centers in their area to find out where cryosurgery is being used.

Chapter 13

Prostate Seed Implants

Radioactive seed implantation for early stage prostate cancer can significantly impair a patient's quality of life, according to a new study by researchers at UCLA's Jonsson Cancer Center.

The findings, published in the March 2000 issue of the *Journal of Urology*, challenge the popular perception that prostate cancer patients who undergo radioactive seed implantation, called brachytherapy, experience better quality of life than patients who undergo radical prostatectomy, or surgery to remove the prostate gland.

Within three to 17 months after finishing treatment, patients in this retrospective study completed questionnaires about their emotional and social functions and physical strength and dexterity, as well as urinary, bowel and sexual functions. Researchers compared quality of life in 48 prostate cancer patients who received seed implants, with or without external beam radiation, with quality of life in 74 patients who underwent surgery.

"Many physicians and patients assume that seed implantation will not have a significant impact on quality of life, but according to our study, that's not true. The effects of seed implantation on a patient's sexual, urinary and bowel function can be significant and patients need to be aware of this when they're considering treatment options," said Dr. Robert Reiter, co-author of the journal article, associate director of the

From "Prostate Seed Implants Impair Quality of Life," by Kambra McConnel, *Daily University Science News,* March 7, 2000, © 2000 UniSci; reprinted with permission from the publisher and authors.

Prostate Program Area at UCLA's Jonsson Cancer Center and an assistant professor of urology at the UCLA School of Medicine.

Although men in the seed implant and surgery groups experienced similar quality of life in terms of physical strength and dexterity and emotional and social functions, the researchers were surprised to find that, on average, patients who underwent seed implantation had significantly more problems with bowel and urinary functions, such as bleeding, diarrhea, burning, and urinating too frequently or too slowly, than men who had surgery.

"We also were surprised to see that patients in the seed implant groups experienced impotence at rates similar to patients in the surgery group," said Dr. Mark Litwin, co-author of the journal article, a researcher at UCLA's Jonsson Cancer Center and an associate professor of Urology at the UCLA School of Medicine. "This finding contradicts previous suggestions that as many as 75 percent of patients who undergo seed implants maintain their potency after treatment. However, the earlier studies were based primarily on physicians' reports, whereas our study relied on patients' self-assessments."

On average, men in the surgery group experienced worse incontinence than those who received seed implants, although men in the seed implant groups reported frequent bouts of incontinence.

In addition to comparing prostate cancer patients who received seed implants with those who underwent surgery, the study for the first time compared quality of life in patients who received seed implants alone with those who received seed implants and external-beam radiation. For about 25 percent of patients with aggressive prostate cancer, external beam radiation is an important part of their treatment because seed implants alone cannot effectively curb their disease.

"Patients need to know that they are more likely to experience worse quality of life in all categories if they undergo seed implantation plus external beam radiation instead of seed implantation alone," Litwin said.

Quality of life has become an increasingly important issue in treatment selection because no single treatment option for prostate cancer has clearly demonstrated a survival advantage, Reiter said.

"The bottom line is that all prostate cancer treatments affect a patient's quality of life, and men need to discuss this fact openly and honestly with their physicians before they decide which particular treatment option is best for them," Reiter said.

UCLA researchers are planning future studies to further investigate quality of life in prostate cancer patients.

Chapter 14

Radiotherapy

Radiotherapy, also called radiation therapy, is the treatment of cancer and other diseases with ionizing radiation. Ionizing radiation deposits energy that injures or destroys cells in the area being treated (the "target tissue") by damaging their genetic material, making it impossible for these cells to continue to grow. Although radiation damages both cancer cells and normal cells, normal cells are better able to repair themselves and function properly. As a result, radiotherapy is more harmful to tumors than normal tissue. Radiotherapy may be used to treat localized solid tumors, such as cancers of the skin, tongue, larynx, brain, breast, or uterine cervix. It can also be used to treat lymphoma (cancer of the immune system).

Radiation used in medical treatment comes in two general forms. The most common form is photon-based energy. Photons are the fundamental units of wave energy such as visible light, X-rays, and gamma rays. X-rays were the first form of photon radiation to be used to treat cancer. Depending on the amount of energy they possess, the rays can be used to destroy cancer cells on the surface of or deeper in the body. The higher the energy of the x-ray beam, the deeper the x-rays can go into the target tissue. Linear accelerators and betatrons are machines that produce x-rays of increasingly greater energy. The use of machines to focus radiation (such as x-rays) on a cancer site is called external beam radiotherapy.

National Cancer Institute (NCI), 1992. Reviewed and updated in May 2001 by Dr. David A. Cooke, MD, Diplomate, American Board of Internal Medicine.

Gamma rays are another form of photons used in radiotherapy. Gamma rays are produced spontaneously as certain elements (such as radium, uranium, and cobalt 60) release radiation as they decompose, or decay. Each element decays at a specific rate and gives off energy in the form of gamma rays and other particles. X-rays and gamma rays have the same effect on cancer cells, but differ in terms of depth of penetration and dose requirements.

Another technique for delivering radiation to cancer cells is to place radioactive implants directly in a tumor or body cavity. This is called internal radiotherapy. (Brachytherapy, interstitial irradiation, and intracavitary irradiation are types of internal radiotherapy.) In this treatment, the radiation dose is concentrated in a small area, and the patient stays in the hospital for a few days. Internal radiotherapy is frequently used for cancers of the tongue, uterus, and cervix. It is also gaining popularity for use against prostate cancer.

Several new approaches to radiation therapy are being evaluated to determine their effectiveness in treating cancer. One such technique is intraoperative irradiation, in which a large dose of external radiation is directed at the tumor and surrounding tissue during surgery.

Another investigational approach is particle beam radiation therapy. This type of therapy differs from photon radiotherapy in that it involves the use of fast-moving subatomic particles to treat localized cancers. A very sophisticated machine is needed to produce and accelerate the particles required for this procedure. Some particles (neutrons, pions, and heavy ions) deposit more energy along the path they take through tissue than do x-rays or gamma rays, thus causing more damage to the cells they hit. This type of radiation is often referred to as high linear energy transfer (high LET) radiation.

Scientists also are looking for ways to increase the effectiveness of radiation therapy. Two types of investigational drugs are being studied for their effect on cells undergoing radiation. Radiosensitizers make the tumor cells more likely to be damaged, and radioprotectors protect normal tissues from the effects of radiation. Hyperthermia, the use of heat, is also being studied for its effectiveness in sensitizing tissue to radiation.

Other recent radiotherapy research has focused on the use of radiolabeled antibodies to deliver doses of radiation directly to the cancer site (radioimmunotherapy). Antibodies are highly specific proteins that are made by the body in response to the presence of antigens (substances recognized as foreign by the immune system). Some tumor cells contain specific antigens that trigger the production of tumor-specific antibodies. Large quantities of these antibodies can be made in the laboratory and attached to radioactive substances (a process known as radiolabeling). Once injected into the body, the antibodies actively seek out the cancer cells, which are destroyed by the cell-killing (cytotoxic) action of the radiation. This approach can minimize the risk of radiation damage to healthy cells. The success of this technique will depend upon both the identification of appropriate radioactive substances and determination of the safe and effective dose of radiation that can be delivered in this way. This form of therapy is still limited to research trials, however.

Radiation therapy may be used alone or in combination with chemotherapy or surgery. Like all forms of cancer treatment, radiation therapy can have side effects. While every effort is made to precisely target cancer cells, some normal cells are also damaged by the radiation. This damage to normal tissue is responsible for the side effects that may occur with radiotherapy. Most side effects are local, occurring in areas the radiation beams pass through. These include loss of hair in the area being treated, skin irritation, and change in skin color or texture. Effects may be temporary or permanent. Fatigue may also occur with radiation therapy, for reasons which are less well understood than local effects.

Chapter 15

Biological Therapy

Biological Therapies: Using the Immune System to Treat Cancer

Biological therapy (sometimes called immunotherapy, biotherapy, or biological response modifier therapy) is a relatively new addition to the family of cancer treatments that also includes surgery, chemotherapy, and radiation therapy. Biological therapies use the body's immune system, either directly or indirectly, to fight cancer or to lessen the side effects that may be caused by some cancer treatments.

The immune system is a complex network of cells and organs that work together to defend the body against attacks by "foreign," or "nonself," invaders. This network is one of the body's main defenses against disease. It works against disease, including cancer, in a variety of ways. For example, the immune system may recognize the difference between healthy cells and cancer cells in the body and work to eliminate those that become cancerous.

Cancer may develop when the immune system breaks down or is not functioning adequately. Biological therapies are designed to repair, stimulate, or enhance the immune system's responses. Immune system cells include the following:

- **Lymphocytes** are a type of white blood cell found in the blood and many other parts of the body. Types of lymphocytes include B cells, T cells, and Natural Killer cells.

CancerNet, National Cancer Institute (NCI), 2000.

113

B cells (B lymphocytes) mature into plasma cells that secrete antibodies (immunoglobulins), the proteins that recognize and attach to foreign substances known as antigens. Each type of B cell makes one specific antibody, which recognizes one specific antigen.

T cells (T lymphocytes) directly attack infected, foreign, or cancerous cells. T cells also regulate the immune response by signaling other immune system defenders. T cells work primarily by producing proteins called lymphokines.

Natural Killer cells (NK cells) produce powerful chemical substances that bind to and kill any foreign invader. They attack without first having to recognize a specific antigen.

- **Monocytes** are white blood cells that can swallow and digest microscopic organisms and particles in a process known as phagocytosis. Monocytes can also travel into tissue and become macrophages, or "big eaters."

Cells in the immune system secrete two types of proteins: antibodies and cytokines. Antibodies respond to antigens by latching on to, or binding with, the antigens. Specific antibodies match specific antigens, fitting together much the way a key fits a lock. Cytokines are substances produced by some immune system cells to communicate with other cells. Types of cytokines include lymphokines, interferons, interleukins, and colony-stimulating factors.

Biological Response Modifiers

Some antibodies, cytokines, and other immune system substances can be produced in the laboratory for use in cancer treatment. These substances are often called biological response modifiers (BRMs). They alter the interaction between the body's immune defenses and cancer cells to boost, direct, or restore the body's ability to fight the disease. BRMs include interferons, interleukins, colony-stimulating factors, monoclonal antibodies, and vaccines.

Researchers continue to discover new BRMs, learn more about how they function, and develop ways to use them in cancer therapy. Biological therapies may be used to:

- Stop, control, or suppress processes that permit cancer growth;

- Make cancer cells more recognizable, and therefore more susceptible, to destruction by the immune system;

- Boost the killing power of immune system cells, such as T cells, NK cells, and acrophages;

- Alter cancer cells' growth patterns to promote behavior like that of healthy cells;

- Block or reverse the process that changes a normal cell or a precancerous cell into a cancerous cell;

- Enhance the body's ability to repair or replace normal cells damaged or destroyed by other forms of cancer treatment, such as chemotherapy or radiation; and

- Prevent cancer cells from spreading to other parts of the body.

Some BRMs are a standard part of treatment for certain types of cancer, while others are being studied in clinical trials (research studies with patients). BRMs are being used alone or in combination with each other. They are also being used with other treatments, such as radiation therapy and chemotherapy.

Interferons (IFN)

Interferons are types of cytokines that occur naturally in the body. They were the first cytokines produced in the laboratory for use as BRMs. There are three major types of interferons—interferon alpha, interferon beta, and interferon gamma; interferon alpha is the type most widely used in cancer treatment.

Researchers have found that interferons can improve the way a cancer patient's immune system acts against cancer cells. In addition, interferons may act directly on cancer cells by slowing their growth or promoting their development into cells with more normal behavior. Researchers believe that some interferons may also stimulate NK cells, T cells, and macrophages, boosting the immune system's anticancer function.

The U.S. Food and Drug Administration (FDA) has approved the use of interferon alpha for the treatment of certain types of cancer, including hairy cell leukemia, melanoma, chronic myeloid leukemia, and AIDS-related Kaposi's sarcoma. Studies have shown that interferon alpha may also be effective in treating other cancers such as metastatic kidney cancer and non-Hodgkin's lymphoma. Researchers are exploring combinations of interferon alpha and other BRMs or chemotherapy in clinical trials to treat a number of cancers.

Interleukins (IL)

Like interferons, interleukins are cytokines that occur naturally in the body and can be made in the laboratory. Many interleukins have been identified; interleukin-2 (IL-2 or aldesleukin) has been the most widely studied in cancer treatment. IL-2 stimulates the growth and activity of many immune cells, such as lymphocytes, that can destroy cancer cells. The FDA has approved IL-2 for the treatment of metastatic kidney cancer and metastatic melanoma.

Researchers continue to study the benefits of interleukins to treat a number of other cancers, including colorectal, ovarian, lung, brain, breast, prostate, some leukemias, and some lymphomas.

Colony-Stimulating Factors (CSFs)

Colony-stimulating factors (CSFs) (sometimes called hematopoietic growth factors) usually do not directly affect tumor cells; rather, they encourage bone marrow cells to divide and develop into white blood cells, platelets, and red blood cells. Bone marrow is critical to the body's immune system because it is the source of all blood cells.

The CSFs' stimulation of the immune system may benefit patients undergoing cancer treatment. Because anticancer drugs can damage the body's ability to make white blood cells, red blood cells, and platelets, patients receiving anticancer drugs have an increased risk of developing infections, becoming anemic, and bleeding more easily. By using CSFs to stimulate blood cell production, doctors can increase the doses of anticancer drugs without increasing the risk of infection or the need for transfusion with blood products. As a result, researchers have found CSFs particularly useful when combined with high-dose chemotherapy.

Some examples of CSFs and their use in cancer therapy are as follows:

- G-CSF (filgrastim) and GM-CSF (sargramostim) can increase the number of white blood cells, thereby reducing the risk of infection in patients receiving chemotherapy. G-CSF and GM-CSF can also stimulate the production of stem cells in preparation for stem cell or bone marrow transplants;

- Erythropoietin can increase the number of red blood cells and reduce the need for transfusions in patients receiving chemotherapy; and

- Oprelvekin can reduce the need for platelet transfusions in patients receiving chemotherapy.

Researchers are studying CSFs in clinical trials to treat some types of leukemia, metastatic colorectal cancer, melanoma, lung cancer, and other types of cancer.

Monoclonal Antibodies (MOABs)

Researchers are evaluating the effectiveness of certain antibodies made in the laboratory called monoclonal antibodies (MOABs or MoABs). These antibodies are produced by a single type of cell and are specific for a particular antigen. Researchers are examining ways to create MOABs specific to the antigens found on the surface of the cancer cell being treated.

MOABs are made by injecting human cancer cells into mice so that their immune systems will make antibodies against these cancer cells. The mouse cells producing the antibodies are then removed and fused with laboratory-grown cells to create "hybrid" cells called hybridomas.

Hybridomas can indefinitely produce large quantities of these pure antibodies, or MOABs. MOABs may be used in cancer treatment in a number of ways:

- MOABs that react with specific types of cancer may enhance a patient's immune response to the cancer.

- MOABs can be programmed to act against cell growth factors, thus interfering with the growth of cancer cells.

- MOABs may be linked to anticancer drugs, radioisotopes (radioactive substances), other BRMs, or other toxins. When the antibodies latch onto cancer cells, they deliver these poisons directly to the tumor, helping to destroy it.

- MOABs may help destroy cancer cells in bone marrow that has been removed from a patient in preparation for a bone marrow transplant.

- MOABs carrying radioisotopes may also prove useful in diagnosing certain cancers, such as colorectal, ovarian, and prostate.

Rituxan-R (rituximab) and Herceptin-R (trastuzumab) are two monoclonal antibodies approved by the FDA. Rituxan is used for the treatment of B-cell non-Hodgkin's lymphoma that has returned after a period of improvement or has not responded to chemotherapy. Herceptin is used to treat metastatic breast cancer in patients with tumors that produce excess amounts of a protein called HER-2. (Approximately 30 percent of breast cancer tumors produce excess amounts of HER-2.) Researchers are testing MOABs in clinical trials to treat lymphomas, leukemias, colorectal cancer, lung cancer, brain tumors, prostate cancer, and other types of cancer.

Cancer Vaccines

Cancer vaccines are another form of biological therapy currently under study. Vaccines for infectious diseases, such as measles, mumps, and tetanus, are effective because they expose the immune system to weakened versions of the disease. This exposure causes the immune system to respond by producing antibodies. Once the immune system has created antibodies, some of the activated immune cells remember the exposure. Therefore, the next time the same antigen enters the body, the immune system can respond more readily to destroy it.

For cancer treatment, researchers are developing vaccines that may encourage the immune system to recognize cancer cells. These vaccines may help the body reject tumors and prevent cancer from recurring. In contrast to vaccines against infectious diseases, cancer vaccines are designed to be injected after the disease is diagnosed, rather than before it develops. Researchers are also investigating ways that cancer vaccines can be used in combination with other BRMs. Cancer vaccines are being studied in the treatment of many types of cancer, including melanoma, lymphomas, and cancers of the kidney, breast, ovaries, prostate, colon, and rectum.

Side Effects

Like other forms of cancer treatment, biological therapies can cause a number of side effects, which can vary widely from patient to patient. Rashes or swelling may develop at the site where the BRMs are injected. Several BRMs, including interferons and interleukins, may cause flu-like symptoms including fever, chills, nausea, vomiting, and appetite loss. Fatigue is another common side effect of BRMs. Blood pressure may also be affected. The side effects of IL-2 can often be severe, depending on the dosage given. Patients need to be closely monitored during treatment. Side effects of CSFs may include bone pain, fatigue, fever, and appetite loss. The side effects of MOABs vary, and serious allergic reactions may occur. Cancer vaccines can cause muscle aches and fever.

Chapter 16

Angiogenesis Inhibitors in the Treatment of Cancer

Angiogenesis means the formation of new blood vessels. Angiogenesis is a process controlled by certain chemicals produced in the body. These chemicals stimulate cells to repair damaged blood vessels or form new ones. Other chemicals, called angiogenesis inhibitors, signal the process to stop.

Angiogenesis plays an important role in the growth and spread of cancer. New blood vessels "feed" the cancer cells with oxygen and nutrients, allowing these cells to grow, invade nearby tissue, spread to other parts of the body, and form new colonies of cancer cells.

Because cancer cannot grow or spread without the formation of new blood vessels, scientists are trying to find ways to stop angiogenesis. They are studying natural and synthetic angiogenesis inhibitors, also called anti-angiogenesis agents, in the hope that these chemicals will prevent the growth of cancer by blocking the formation of new blood vessels. In animal studies, angiogenesis inhibitors have successfully stopped the formation of new blood vessels, causing the cancer to shrink and die.

Whether angiogenesis inhibitors will be effective against cancer in humans is not yet known. Various angiogenesis inhibitors are currently being evaluated in clinical trials (research studies in humans). These studies include patients with cancers of the breast, prostate, brain, pancreas, lung, stomach, ovary, and cervix; some leukemias and lymphomas; and AIDS-related Kaposi's sarcoma. If the results of

CancerNet, National Cancer Institute (NCI), 1998.

clinical trials show that angiogenesis inhibitors are both safe and effective in treating cancer in humans, these agents may be approved by the Food and Drug Administration (FDA) and made available for widespread use. The process of producing and testing angiogenesis inhibitors is likely to take several years.

Detailed information about ongoing clinical trials evaluating angiogenesis inhibitors and other promising new treatments is available from the Cancer Information Service (CIS). The CIS, a national information and education network, is a free public service of the National Cancer Institute (NCI), the Nation's primary agency for cancer research. The CIS meets the information needs of patients, the public, and health professionals. The toll-free phone number is 1-800-4-CANCER (1-800-422-6237). For callers with TTY equipment, the number is 1-800-332-8615. The NCI's clinical trials website also provides a listing of NCI-sponsored clinical trials at http://cancertrials. nci.nih.gov on the Internet.

Chapter 17

Selenium Supplements for Prevention of Prostate Cancer

Selenium Lowers Incidence of Lung, Colorectal, and Prostate Cancers

A 10-year cancer prevention trial suggests that dietary supplements of the trace element selenium may significantly lower the incidence of prostate, colorectal, and lung cancers in people with a history of skin cancer. The supplements did not, however, affect the incidence of basal or squamous cell cancers of the skin, the original hypothesis of the study. The results are published in the 12/25/96 issue of the *Journal of the American Medical Association*. The study is titled: "Effects of Selenium Supplementation for Cancer Prevention in Patients with Carcinoma of the Skin." The authors are Larry C. Clark, Gerald F. Combs Jr., Bruce W. Turnbull, Elizabeth H. Slate, Daniel K. Chalker, James Chow, Loretta S. Davis, Renee A. Glover, Gloria F. Graham, Earl G. Gross, Arnon Krongrad, Jack Lesher, H. Kim Park, Beverly B. Sanders Jr., Cameron L. Smith, J. Richard Taylor.

The study began in 1983 and included a total of 1,312 skin cancer patients with a mean age of 63 seen at seven dermatology clinics in the eastern United States. At that time, the primary purpose of the study was to see if dietary supplements of selenium could lower the incidence of basal cell or squamous cell skin cancers. In 1990, secondary end points, including incidence of the most commonly occurring cancers, lung, prostate, and colorectal were added.

Cancer Facts, National Cancer Institute (NCI), 1997.

"The results of this study are exciting because they show the cancer prevention potential of a nutritional supplement to a normal diet," said Larry C. Clark, Ph.D., MPH, associate professor of epidemiology at the Arizona Cancer Center in Tucson, Ariz., and principal investigator of the study. "The study needs to be repeated in other populations before a public health recommendation can be made for selenium supplementation."

Patients in the double-blinded (neither patients nor doctors knew who was receiving the intervention), randomized study took a tablet containing 200 micrograms (ug) of selenium as brewer's yeast, or placebo, daily for 4.5 years and were followed for an additional 6.4 years. Three-quarters of the patients were men. The trial ended in January 1996, two years before the planned end of the trial.

American diets generally include enough grain, meat, and fish, the primary sources of selenium, to meet the recommended dietary allowance (RDA), 70 ug/day for men and 55 ug/day for women. (Although the EPA established a reference dose, 350 ug/day, as a measure of the maximum safe intake, the human toxicity levels for selenium have not been definitely established.) The study population, however, was from a region of the eastern United States with relatively low selenium levels in soils and crops, and before treatment had a mean plasma selenium concentration in the lower range of the U.S. levels. The supplements increased the plasma concentration by 67 percent and the average daily intakes by 3-fold. The higher plasma concentrations were reached within six to nine months of supplementation and were maintained throughout the trial, although a small decline was seen over the course of the trial.

The results of the study showed that total cancer incidence was significantly lower in the selenium group than in the placebo group (77 cases versus 119), as was the incidence of some site-specific cancers: the selenium group had fewer prostate cancers (13 versus 35), fewer colorectal cancers (8 versus 19), and fewer lung cancers (17 versus 31). These differences were statistically significant. The number of cases at other sites were insufficient for a valid analysis.

The results also showed that over-all mortality was 17 percent less in the selenium versus the control group (108 versus 129) with this difference largely due to a 50 percent reduction in cancer deaths (29 versus 57). Lung cancer deaths were lower in the selenium-treatment group than in the placebo (12 versus 26). The number of deaths for other cancers were insufficient for meaningful statistical analysis. There was no significant difference between the two treatment groups for other causes of death.

Peter Greenwald, M.D., director of the National Cancer Institutes Division of Cancer Prevention and Control commented, "These results are interesting for several reasons. First, there was no detectable increase in adverse effects from the supplementation which is very important to know for future trials. Secondly, beneficial effects were seen for three major cancers." "Having said all that," he added, "we need to be cautious." Greenwald noted that the study population was relatively small and consisted of people who live in low-selenium regions and are at high risk for non-melanoma skin cancer. The lower cancer rates were found for cancers that were secondary, not primary study endpoints. The work, he believes, needs to be confirmed in a larger population more representative of the U.S.

Selenium soil levels were first associated inversely with cancer mortality in the late 1960s. Similar results were found in prospective studies which measured selenium status by several methods; soil, blood, nails, hair. Some studies have also found inverse associations with the incidence of cancers of the lung, colon, bladder, rectum, breast, pancreas, and ovary. However, several studies have shown no association between selenium status and cancer and a few have shown a direct association—cancer risk increased with selenium status.

In animals, selenium administration has been shown to have anti-tumor activity, but at levels several times greater than the nutritional needs. Likewise, in tissue culture experiments, supplementation of cultured tumor cells with selenium at much higher doses than the cells normally require, has been shown to inhibit tumor growth and stimulate apoptosis, programmed cell death. Three human intervention studies with selenium have had various outcomes. The low soil selenium content in Finland led the Finnish government to begin adding selenium to fertilizers in 1984 with an eye towards reducing cancer risk and cardiovascular disease. No significant effects on cancer incidence have been seen to date in the Finnish population of four million.

Two additional human intervention trials took place in Linxian, China from 1985-1991. In one trial, a daily supplement containing 50 ug selenium plus three other minerals and vitamins, had no effect on the high incidence of esophageal cancer or total cancer incidence or mortality. The second and largest trial showed a significant reduction in stomach cancer incidence (16 percent) and stomach cancer mortality (21 percent) using a daily mixture of antioxidants—one component of which was selenium.

The current study is the first double-blinded cancer prevention trial to test whether a nutritional supplement of selenium alone can reduce cancer risk. Participating dermatology clinics were located in Augusta, GA; Macon, GA; Columbia, S.C.; Miami, FLA; Wilson, N.C.; Greenville, N.C.; and Newington, Conn.

Greenwald commented on the possibility of future prevention trials. "This study highlights the value of clinical trials in cancer prevention. The interesting observation of a possible benefit of selenium needs to be assessed in a larger, more definitive trial."

Chapter 18

Alternative Medicine

Complementary and alternative medicine (CAM)—also referred to as integrative medicine—includes a broad range of healing philosophies, approaches, and therapies. A therapy is generally called complementary when it is used in addition to conventional treatments; it is often called alternative when it is used instead of conventional treatment. (Conventional treatments are those that are widely accepted and practiced by the mainstream medical community.) Depending on how they are used, some therapies can be considered either complementary or alternative.

Complementary and alternative therapies are used in an effort to prevent illness, reduce stress, prevent or reduce side effects and symptoms, or control or cure disease. Some commonly used methods of complementary or alternative therapy include mind/body control interventions such as visualization or relaxation, manual healing including acupressure and massage, homeopathy, vitamins or herbal products, and acupuncture.

Following are a series of frequently asked questions and answers about complementary and alternative medicine.

Are complementary and alternative cancer therapies widely used?

Although there are few studies on the use of complementary and alternative therapies for cancer, one large-scale study found that the

CancerNet, National Cancer Institute (NCI), 1999.

127

percentage of cancer patients in the United States using these therapies was nine percent overall (Lerner and Kennedy, 1992).

Can complementary and alternative medicine be evaluated using the same methods used in conventional medicine?

Scientific evaluation is important in understanding if and when complementary and alternative therapies work. A number of medical centers are evaluating complementary and alternative therapies by developing scientific studies to test them.

Conventional approaches to cancer treatment have generally been studied for safety and effectiveness through a rigorous scientific process, including clinical trials with large numbers of patients. Often, less is known about the safety and effectiveness of complementary and alternative methods. Some of these complementary and alternative therapies have not undergone rigorous evaluation. Others, once considered unorthodox, are finding a place in cancer treatment—not as cures, but as complementary therapies that may help patients feel better and recover faster. One example is acupuncture. According to a panel of experts at a National Institutes of Health Consensus Conference in November 1997, acupuncture has been found to be effective in the management of chemotherapy-associated nausea and vomiting and in controlling pain associated with surgery. Some approaches, such as laetrile, have been studied and found ineffective or potentially harmful.

What should patients do when considering complementary and alternative therapies?

Cancer patients considering complementary and alternative medicine should discuss this decision with their doctor or nurse, as they would any therapeutic approach, because some complementary and alternative therapies may interfere with their standard treatment or may be harmful when used with conventional treatment.

When considering complementary and alternative therapies, what questions should patients ask their health care provider?

- What benefits can be expected from this therapy?
- What are the risks associated with this therapy?
- Do the known benefits outweigh the risks?

- What side effects can be expected?
- Will the therapy interfere with conventional treatment?
- Will the therapy be covered by health insurance?

How can patients and their health care providers learn more about complementary and alternative therapies?

Patients and their doctor or nurse can learn about complementary and alternative therapies from the following Government agencies:

The NIH National Center for Complementary and Alternative Medicine

(NCCAM) facilitates research and evaluation of complementary and alternative practices and has information about a variety of methods.

NCCAM Clearinghouse
Post Office Box 8218
Silver Spring, MD 20907-8218
Toll Free: 888-644-6226
TTY/TDY: 888-644-6226 (toll free)
Internet: http://nccam.nih.gov
E-Mail: nccam-info@nih.gov

The Food and Drug Administration (FDA)

FDA regulates drugs and medical devices to ensure that they are safe and effective.

Food and Drug Administration
5600 Fishers Lane
Rockville, MD 20857
Telephone: 888-463-6332 (toll free)
Internet: http://www.fda.gov

References

Cassileth, B., Chapman, C., Alternative and Complementary Cancer Therapies. *Cancer* 1996; 77(6):1026-1033.

Jacobs, J., Unproven Alternative Methods of Cancer Treatment. In: DeVita, Hellman, Rosenberg, editors. *Cancer: Principles and Practice of Oncology. 5th edition.* Philadelphia: Lippincott-Raven Publishers; 1997. 2993-3001.

Lerner, I.J., Kennedy, B.J., The Prevalence of Questionable Methods of Cancer Treatment in the United States. *CA-A Cancer Journal* 1992;42:181-191.

Nelson, W., Alternative Cancer Treatments. *Highlights in Oncology Practice* 1998; 15(4):85-93.

Chapter 19

Caring for Your Health and Feelings after Cancer Treatment

What You Can Expect

After you have been treated for cancer, you will have two ongoing health needs. First, you'll want to take the health steps that doctors suggest for anyone your age. Second, you'll have special needs for caring for your body based on your type of cancer, treatment, and current state of health.

Other long-term health needs for cancer survivors differ from person to person. In addition to regular checkups, you may need rehabilitation or home care. Some survivors may need help in dealing with emotional or sexual problems, while others may seek pain control therapy. And more cancer treatment sometimes occurs. To get a good picture of your individual needs, ask your doctor. He or she can let you know what you need to do this year—and in the future—to take care of your health. The following stories highlight some of the most common issues for cancer survivors.

- "I had expected that leaving the hospital after cancer treatment would be the happiest day of my life. When that time came, though, I was actually more afraid than happy. I felt very alone, and I missed the support of being watched over and cared for by the medical team. My social worker said that this was a common reaction, but I remember that my family had a hard time understanding it."

  —Jack C.

CancerNet, National Cancer Institute (NCI), 2000.

131

- "In the first couple of years after my recovery, the thing I hated most was going in for my checkups. Just seeing the hospital again reminded me of a part of my life I'd rather have forgotten. I had an almost physical reaction to the sounds and smells of the place. But more than that, those visits reminded me that I'd been sick and that my cancer might recur. In my daily life, I'd kept those thoughts out of my mind.

  Fortunately, it's better now. Maybe I've just gotten used to the routine, and I also understand how important these checkups are to my health."

  —Janet V.

- "I find I walk a fine line between watching for signs of recurrence or long-term effects of my radiation therapy and going overboard. I never used to be like this, but it's hard not to be scared by changes that might mean problems. My first doctor was not very sympathetic about my concerns, so I found another doctor who is. She understands, and she doesn't tell me 'it's all in your head.' "

  —Louise F.

- "I'm in a support group for cancer survivors, and we have people with all kinds of cancers who've made all kinds of adjustments: living with artificial limbs, ostomies, breast changes, energy loss, chronic pain. But we all have one thing in common. At one time or another we each have been so angry that this happened to us. Before I joined the group, my anger was having as much of a negative effect on my life as my disability. Talking about it, and seeing how others cope, helped me put things in perspective."

  —Sacha R.

- "When I think about my cancer treatment, I almost feel like it began when I left the hospital after surgery. Much of my care took place at home—for a while my room looked like a hospital. Now I'm back to the hospital some times for radiation therapy to control my pain. I'm getting used to the fact that my cancer is more like a lifelong, chronic disease that I need to manage than something the doctors can 'cure' once and for all."

  —Irene L.

- "My family wonders if it's a waste of time and money for me to get yearly checkups for the colon cancer I had 15 years ago. But I feel that I'm doing something important for my health."

—Rhea S.

Basics of Health Care for Cancer Survivors

- Get regular checkups. In general, people who have been treated for cancer return regularly to the doctor every 3-4 months at first, and once or twice a year later on. Ask your doctor how often you should be rechecked.

- Be alert to signs of a possible return of cancer and long-term effects of treatment. Ask your doctor to explain what symptoms should be watched.

- Get tested as needed for other cancers. Your doctor can tell you how often you should have tests to detect breast cancer and colon cancer. With early detection, these cancers often can be controlled.

- Have good health habits: Eating right and getting enough sleep and exercise will help you feel better.

Tips for Managing Your Care

- Keep accurate, up-to-date records of all the medical care you receive for cancer and other conditions. Future decisions about your care may depend on how you have been treated in the past. If you move or go to several different doctors, no one but you will have your complete history.

- Do things you enjoy, even if you don't feel perfect. Pleasure can be a powerful tool for health.

- Work as a partner with your doctors and other health professionals in your continuing care. When you first were treated for cancer, you may have taken an active part in making decisions about your care. The same active role can help you take control of your long term health needs. The two main steps are to ask questions and give information to your caregivers.

Ask Questions

You need information to carry out your role in managing your care. These facts are as important to quality of care as any other aspect of treatment. With this in mind, no question you have about your care is "dumb." Many people bring a tape recorder, take notes, or ask a friend along to help them remember everything that's said. It is also a good idea to bring a list of questions when you visit your doctor. The following are some questions you may want to ask:

- How often should I have a checkup?

- What are the signs of cancer's return or of long-term effects?

- How likely are they to occur?

- What changes might I see that are not danger signs?

- What kind of diet should I have?

- What are my treatment options for handling chronic pain, the return of cancer, the long-term effects of therapy?

- What is the best way to talk to you about my concerns? (By phone? At a special appointment? At a regular visit scheduled in advance to run longer?)

- Who else is available to talk with me about specific problems (e.g. sexual concerns, care instructions, general fitness)?

Give Information

Doctors need to know key facts about you to prescribe the best treatments and help keep you involved in your care. Tell them:

- What medicines you now are taking for all conditions (including over-the-counter medicines such as aspirin or laxatives). Doctors need this information to avoid problems when they give you a new medicine.

- About fears or concerns you have, especially those that might be keeping you from following treatment. Talking openly may help solve the problem.

- About changes in your lifestyle. Even changes that seem minor could affect your treatment. For example, if you quit smoking you may need a different dose of some medicines.

- How you are feeling. Include danger signs you may have noticed as well as any other changes that may be worrying you.

- About problems you may have and how much the doctor tells you about your cancer. You have a right to hear as much or as little information as you wish.

Options for Coping with Body Changes

Get help if you need it.

- Ask your nurse or the social worker at your hospital about homemaker services, home health services, seminars and classes, rides to the hospital, and other community aid. Find out how to use special tools to over come disability or discomfort.

- Mechanical aids can replace many lost functions. Talk to your rehabilitation professional. Learn from others who have the same problem.

- Ask your local cancer support organization, social worker, or doctor's office staff to put you in touch with other survivors. They can give you practical tips to make your new situation easier. Find ways to meet your needs for intimacy.

- Most survivors of any cancer can still enjoy sexual touching and sexual closeness.

- Talk to your doctor, nurse, or therapist to learn proven ideas for solving problems. Focus on your best features.

- Make the most of them with makeup, clothes, or accessories. Feel good about yourself. Find new shopping sources for products that help you look better.

- Ask your local cancer support organization, your social worker, and other survivors for ideas and addresses.

Looking Good

Some people who've had cancer treatment must adjust to a new body image. Cosmetic aids, such as artificial limbs or wigs, may help boost self-confidence as well as provide physical comfort. After a mastectomy, for example, a woman may wear a breast form to give shape and weight to where her breast was removed. Patients who lose hair due to chemotherapy may wear wigs.

- If you plan to buy a cosmetic aid, you may want to contact your local American Cancer Society unit, which may have a list of stores that sell them. The unit also may maintain a "wig bank," a collection of wigs that are given free of charge to cancer patients. Or call the Cancer Information Service at 1-800-4-CANCER, which may have a list of local stores that sell the product you need. And check with your insurance company. Some policies cover some cosmetic aids.

Sexual Concerns

Cancer and cancer treatment may affect sexual relationships. Although treatment for cancer sometimes causes sexual problems, often a patient's or partner's feelings about cancer and sex can make a difference. Your doctor, nurse, or social worker may be able to help. They also may be able to help you find a sex therapist who helps couples understand their sexual problems and suggests ways to deal with them.

Taking Care of Your Feelings

What kinds of feelings are "normal"? There is no "right" way to feel; the important thing is to handle your emotions in a way that works for you. Many survivors find that the key for them is talking their feelings out-with family and friends, health professionals, other patients, and counselors such as clergy and psychotherapists.

The following stories show the range of feelings that many cancer survivors have. Each of them is a normal reaction that is often part of the cancer survivor's life.

- "In the first 6 months after my cancer treatment, I saw my cancer more as a threat to my life plans for marriage and a career than I did as a threat to my life. I felt the most depressed and anxious during the first 3 months, but then I started to get back to normal. I say started, because I'm not sure I'm there yet. It's getting better, but I still feel a little off balance."

  —Marcia B.

- "I don't intend to focus on cancer for the rest of my life. I follow my care plan but I don't dwell on the disease or talk about it to others. Some (I suppose) well-meaning people at the office said that my reaction is called denial, and that it is bad for me. I talked about it with the doctor, and he said denial can be positive when it helps you get on with your life. I have my ups and downs like every one else, but I feel good about the way I'm handling my disease."

—Joe K.

- "I have to say that there's been one positive result of my having had cancer. It made me look at the real possibility of my own death, something I had never thought much about before. That made me take a hard look at my life and decide what really mattered to me. As a survivor, I now see every day as a precious gift."

—Vicki W.

- "My cancer treatment ended 10 years ago, but I still get anxious every time I go in for a checkup. The nurse told me that's a common reaction."

—Dave L.

- "I was very surprised at how few of my friends really made the effort to 'be there' for me. I talked to the nurse about this during my last checkup. She said that people often want to help but they don't know how—and they may be embarrassed to ask. So I decided to make the first move with some of the people I cared about most. It was hard, but I think I broke down a wall when I spoke openly about my feelings and my needs. I feel much more in touch and supported now."

—Rhonda L.

- "My cancer has led to some difficult family situations. The hardest thing was learning to adjust to different family roles. My wife went back to work during my recovery, and my teenage daughter had to take care of the house. As I got better, none of us was sure what roles were 'normal' and my daughter especially didn't want any changes that limited her independence. At that point the doctor suggested family therapy. I had my doubts, but seeing the real problems behind the obvious problems made a difference. After we worked through solutions together, I think we're closer now than ever before."

—Ralph Y.

- "The most important source of hope and support for me has been my faith in God. When I face my fears and uncertainties, I know I'm not alone."

  —Frances C.

- "Surviving cancer has been not one condition but many. It was such happiness at the birth of a daughter in the midst of concerns about the future. It was the joy of eating Chinese food for the first time after radiation burns in my esophagus had healed. It has been the anxiety of waiting for test results and the fear that the cancer would recur. It has been having a positive attitude and wanting to strangle the people who told me that was all it would take."

  —Frank T.

- "People have recovered from every type of cancer, no matter how gloomy the first reports. Yes, we're all going to die someday of something. But I plan to push that day back as far as I can, and to go out fighting whenever the time comes."

  —Betty R.

Surviving Cancer—Hopeful Trends

- There are over 8 million cancer survivors in America today.

- If lung cancer deaths were excluded, cancer mortality would have declined 14 percent between 1950 and 1990.

- The number of people who have survived cancer for 5 or more years has increased significantly since 1973 for cancers of the colon, stomach, testis, and bladder, and for Hodgkin's disease and leukemia.

- Studies show that for most patients the emotional upset after cancer diagnosis and treatment decreases over time.

Tips for Coping with Survivor Stress

The following tips come from the experiences of survivors in the American Cancer Society's "I Can Cope" program. They are adapted from ideas appearing in a book, *I Can Cope-Staying Healthy with Cancer*, coauthored by the program's cofounder, Judi Johnson.

- Be kind to yourself. Instead of telling yourself you can't do something you should do, focus on what you can do and what you want to do. Instead of telling yourself you look awful, think of ways to make the most of your best features.

- Help others. Reaching out to someone else can reduce the stress caused by brooding.

- Don't be afraid to say no. Polite but firm refusals help you stay in control of your life.

- Talk about your concerns. It's the best way to release them.

- Learn to pace yourself. Stop before you get tired.

- Give in sometimes. Not every argument is worth winning.

- Get enough exercise. It's a great way to get rid of tension and aggression in a positive way.

- Take time for activities you enjoy, whether it's a hobby, club, or special project.

- Take one thing at a time. If you're feeling overwhelmed, divide your list into manageable parts.

- Set priorities. Don't try to be Superman or Superwoman.

- Solve problems like an expert. First, identify the problem and write it down, so it's clear in your mind. Second, list your options with the pros and cons of each. Third, choose a plan. Fourth, list the steps to accomplish it. Then give yourself a deadline and act. Sometimes just having a plan can reduce the stress of the problem.

- Eat properly.

- Get enough sleep.

- Laugh at least once a day.

Is a Survivors' Group Right for You?

If you answer "yes" to most of the following questions, joining a cancer survivors' group may be a positive step for you.

- Are you comfortable sharing your feelings with others in a similar situation?

- Are you interested in hearing others' feelings about their experiences?

- Could you benefit from the advice of others who have gone through cancer treatment?

- Do you enjoy being part of a group?

- Do you have helpful information or hints to share with others?

- Would reaching out to support other cancer survivors give you satisfaction?

- Would you feel comfortable working with survivors who have different ways of facing forward?

- Are you interested in learning more about cancer and survivor issues?

Options for Getting Emotional Support

Join a cancer survivors' group.

- Ask your doctor, nurse, or social worker about programs available at local hospitals.

- Call your local cancer support organizations, including the American Cancer Society, which may sponsor groups in your area. Check the telephone book for contact information.

Talk to your family and friends.

- Help them understand how they can help you.

- Talk about their needs for support.

Talk to your clergyman or clergywoman.

- Consider professional mental health assistance.

- Consult a psychologist, nurse therapist, clinical social worker, or psychiatrist.

- For marital or family issues, consult a licensed or family therapist.

Work with someone on the medical team to solve problems.

- Get help in dealing with your hospital, clinic, or health maintenance organization.

- Ask about health concerns that cause you stress.

Support yourself.

- Draw on your own strength.

- Read about how others cope. Ask at your local bookstore for accounts by cancer survivors.

Reach out to others.

- Helping others can help you feel stronger and more in control.

- For some people, helping other cancer survivors is a satisfying way to reach out.

Chapter 20

Post-Treatment Concerns: Incontinence, Impotence, and Infertility

Following cancer treatment, a number of post treatment concerns arise. Among them are, incontinence, impotence, and issues related to fertility. This chapter addresses those concerns, and contains helpful information related to these issues.

Urinary Incontinence

Urinary incontinence is the loss of bladder control or the leakage of urine. It can happen to anyone, but is very common in older people. At least 1 out of 10 people age 65 or older suffers from incontinence. It is a condition that rages from mild leakage to uncontrollable and embarrassing wetting. Urinary incontinence is a major health problem because it can lead to disability and dependency.

Many people with incontinence pull away from their family and friends. They try to hide the problem from everyone, even their doctors. The good news is that in most cases urinary incontinence can be treated and controlled, if not cured. The bad news is that caregivers may not know that treatment is a choice. They may think that nursing home care is the only answer for an older person with incontinence.

Text in this chapter is excerpted from "Urinary Incontinence," *Age Page*, National Institute on Aging, 1996; "Sexuality Later in Life," *Age Page*, National Institute on Aging, 1994; and "Fertility After Cancer...Options for Starting a Family," Virtual Hospital, © 1997 University of Iowa; reprinted with permission.

Incontinence does not happen because of aging. It may be caused by changes in your body due to disease. For example, incontinence may be the first and only symptom of a urinary tract infection. Curing the infection may relieve or cure the problem. Some drugs may cause incontinence or make it worse.

If you are having trouble with incontinence, see your doctor. Even if it can't be completely cured, modern products and ways of managing incontinence can ease its discomfort and inconvenience.

Types of Incontinence

The most common types of urinary incontinence are:

• *Stress incontinence* happens when urine leaks during exercise, coughing, sneezing, laughing, lifting heavy objects, or other body movements that put pressure on the bladder. It is the most common type of incontinence and can almost always be cured.

• *Urge incontinence* happens if you can't hold your urine long enough to reach a toilet. Although healthy people can have urge incontinence, it is often found in people who have diabetes, stroke, dementia, Parkinson's disease, or multiple sclerosis. It can also be a warning sign of early bladder cancer. In men, it is often a sign of an enlarged prostate.

• *Overflow incontinence* happens when small amounts of urine leak from a bladder that is always full. In older men, this can occur when the flow of urine from the bladder is blocked. Some people with diabetes also have this problem.

• *Functional incontinence* happens in many older people who have relatively normal urine control but who have a hard time getting to the toilet in time because of arthritis or other crippling disorders.

Diagnosis

The first and most important step in treating incontinence is to see a doctor for a complete medical exam. The doctor will ask for a detailed history of your health and give you a physical exam. The doctor may want to check urine samples. You may be referred to a urologist, a doctor who specializes in diseases of the urinary tract, or to a gynecologist, a specialist in the female reproductive system.

Treatment

Treatment of urinary incontinence should be designed to meet your needs. As a general rule, the least dangerous procedures should be tried first. The many options include:

- Behavioral techniques such as pelvic muscle exercises, biofeedback, and bladder training can help control urination. These techniques can help you sense your bladder filling and help delay voiding until you can reach a toilet.

- A doctor can prescribe medicines to treat incontinence. However, these drugs may cause side effects such as dry mouth, eye problems, or urine buildup.

- Sometimes surgery can improve or cure incontinence if it is caused by a structural problem such as an abnormally positioned bladder or blockage due to an enlarged prostate. Implanting devices that replace or aid the muscles controlling urine flow has been tried in people with incontinence.

Management

If your incontinence cannot be cured, it can be managed in several ways.

- You can get special absorbent underclothing that is no more bulky than normal underwear and can be worn easily under everyday clothing.

- A flexible tube (indwelling catheter) can be put into the urethra (the canal that carries the urine from the bladder) to collect urine in a container. Long-term catheterization—although sometimes necessary—creates many problems, including urinary infections. Men have the choice of an external collecting device. This is fitted over the penis and connected to a drainage bag.

Remember, under a doctor's care, incontinence can be treated and often cured. Even if treatment is not fully successful, careful management can help.

Impotence

Most older people want and are able to enjoy an active, satisfying sex life. Regular sexual activity helps maintain sexual ability. However, over time everyone may notice a slowing of response. This is part of the normal aging process.

Men often notice more distinct changes. It may take longer to get an erection or the erection may not be as firm or as large as in earlier years. The feeling that an ejaculation is about to happen may be shorter. The loss of erection after orgasm may be more rapid or it may take longer before an erection is again possible. Some men may find they need more manual stimulation.

As men get older, impotence seems to increase, especially in men with heart disease, hypertension, and diabetes. Impotence is the loss of ability to achieve and maintain an erection hard enough for sexual intercourse. Talk to your doctor. For many men impotence can be managed and perhaps even reversed.

Effects of Illness or Disability

Prostatectomy is the surgical removal of all or part of the prostate. Sometimes a prostatectomy needs to be done because of an enlarged prostate. This procedure rarely causes impotence. If a radical prostatectomy (removal of prostate gland) is needed, new surgical techniques can save the nerves going to the penis and an erection may still be possible. If your sexuality is important to you, talk to your doctor before surgery to make sure you will be able to lead a fully satisfying sex life. Although illness or disability can affect sexuality, even the most serious conditions shouldn't stop you from having a satisfying sex life.

Other Issues

Heart disease. Many people who have had a heart attack are afraid that having sex will cause another attack. The risk of this is very low. Follow your doctor's advice. Most people can start having sex again 12 to 16 weeks after an attack.

Diabetes. Most men with diabetes do not have problems, but it is one of the few illnesses that can cause impotence. In most cases medical treatment can help.

Stroke. Sexual function is rarely damaged by a stroke and it is unlikely that sexual exertion will cause another stroke. Using different positions or medical devices can help make up for any weakness or paralysis.

Arthritis. Joint pain due to arthritis can limit sexual activity. Surgery and drugs may relieve this pain. In some cases drugs can decrease sexual desire. Exercise, rest, warm baths, and changing the position or timing of sexual activity can be helpful.

Surgery. Most people worry about having any kind of surgery—it is especially troubling when the sex organs are involved. The good news is that most people do return to the kind of sex life they enjoyed before having surgery.

Alcohol. Too much alcohol can reduce potency in men and delay orgasm in women.

Medicines. Antidepressants, tranquilizers, and certain high blood pressure drugs can cause impotence. Some drugs can make it difficult for men to ejaculate. Some drugs reduce a woman's sexual desire. Check with your doctor. She or he can often prescribe a drug without this side effect.

Emotional Concerns

Sexuality is often a delicate balance of emotional and physical issues. How we feel may affect what we are able to do. For example, men may fear impotence will become a more frequent problem as they age. But, if you are too worried about impotence, you can create enough stress to cause it.

Older couples may have the same problems that affect people of any age. But they may also have the added concerns of age, retirement and other lifestyle changes, and illness. These problems can cause sexual difficulties. Talk openly with your doctor or see a therapist. These health professionals can often help.

Fertility

A person is never ready to hear he or she has cancer. The diagnosis of cancer can bring on many emotions as well as questions. Time and careful thought are needed to sort through all the questions you may have about your disease, as well as the treatment and how it affects you.

People diagnosed with cancer are being treated with more intense treatments and living longer. Questions about starting a family may come up. After cancer treatment the chances of having children may be decreased or eliminated due to the effects of treatment. As difficult as it might be, the best time to discuss options for starting a family is at the beginning of your treatment. Questions like "Am I going to live?" and "When do I start treatment?" take priority over "Does my future allow for me to start a family?" Cancer can be a life-threatening illness and may need to be treated as soon as possible, but in many cases it is possible to take the steps needed to plan for future reproduction. Your doctor or health care team will help to guide you in your decisions. Be open and honest with your doctor and nurses about all your concerns and questions, They are there to help meet your needs.

This chapter contains an overview of the normal reproductive system, and describes how different cancer treatments affect your ability to have children.

You may or may not want to have children after cancer treatment, but there is no way to know whether the ability to have children will return to normal or not. Included are options for starting a family after cancer treatment, and how to go about getting assistance. It helps to know what to expect in advance and it may be reassuring to know what options are open to you. There is more to a person's sexuality and intimacy than reproductive issues.

Male Reproductive System

Sperm are made in tiny thread-like tubes (seminiferous tubules) in the testicles. It takes seventy-four days for a sperm cell to mature. The body makes hormones that are needed for sperm to be made. Testosterone is one of the hormones needed for making sperm. The same hormones that are needed in females (follicle stimulating hormone, and luteinizing hormone) are also needed to make sperm. The sperm move from the testicles through a long coiled tube called the epididymis, where they finish growing and then are stored. At the time of release, the sperm is mixed with fluid from the seminal vesicles and prostate gland. This fluid is called semen and helps to nourish and protect the sperm against the acidic environment of the vagina. Semen passes through a tube in the penis to the outside of the body. Urine also passes through this same tube in the penis. During sexual intercourse the semen is ejaculated or released into a woman's vagina near the opening of the uterus (womb), called the cervix. The sperm must swim through the cervix, the uterus and into the fallopian tubes where the fertilization of the egg can happen. When the sperm meets with the fertile egg, the chemicals stored in the head of the sperm will help the sperm to enter the egg. The genetic material (DNA) of the sperm will join with that of the egg and fertilization occurs. This beginning of a baby is called an embryo. In five to seven days the embryo must implant itself in the lining of the uterus, so that it can grow. This is how a pregnancy begins.

Cancer Treatments and How They Affect the Ability to Have Children

The type of cancer you have may change the way your reproductive system works even before you receive treatment. Treatment can also affect your fertility or ability to have children. Following are treatments that may alter your ability to have children.

Chemotherapy

Cancer treatment with chemotherapy may affect your fertility. The effects of chemotherapy for both men and women depend on: your age, the types of drugs, the amounts of the drugs you receive, and how many months your treatment lasts.

In men, chemotherapy can cause a lowered sperm count or even sterility (an inability to father children). The effects on a man's ability to father children may be temporary, or can last for as long as two to four years, or they may be for life. Some method of birth control should be used during treatment. There is a risk of passing on some of the cancer drugs through the semen, so the use of condoms is recommended during treatment.

Sperm banking is an option for some people. Sperm banking should be considered before treatment begins. It is known that we can safely collect sperm samples for sperm banking up to twenty days after the start of chemotherapy. If you are interested in this option, it is important that you discuss this with your doctor at the beginning of your treatment plans.

Radiation Therapy

Radiation to the pelvis or area of the reproductive organs can damage or destroy reproductive tissues and cells. Men may have problems fathering a child when radiation therapy is given to an area that includes the testicles. Radiation can reduce the number of sperm and the ability of the sperm to fertilize an egg. This may be temporary or for life. It is possible for a pregnancy to occur while receiving radiation treatment so it is necessary to use birth control during treatment. It is unclear what harm is done to the sperm and how that would affect a pregnancy. Concerns about birth control measures, as well as lower sperm counts, should be discussed with your doctor. Sperm banking is an option for some people. Sperm banking should be considered before treatment begins. If you are interested in this option it is important that you discuss this with your doctor.

Many cancer patients receive external beam radiation therapy which delivers radiation through the skin.

Surgical Treatment

To understand how surgery may affect a man's ability to father a child, it may help to review the parts of the male anatomy that are involved and what their roles are in reproduction.

For a man to release sperm into a woman's vagina, it is necessary for him to have an erection. For an erection to occur, there needs to be an increased blood flow to the penis causing it to become full and firm. If you have a surgery that blocks or changes the blood flow to your penis, you may have trouble having an erection.

Surgery involving the nerves around the rectum and pelvic floor may also result in the inability to have an erection. If the testicles can still produce sperm and the seminal vesicles can still produce semen, the ability to father a child is still present.

The nerves in the pelvic floor and that surround the abdominal aorta (large blood vessel in the abdomen) are also involved with the control of the valves in the penis that direct the release of sperm and semen. A "dry" ejaculation can occur if there is no semen or if the semen is ejaculated into the bladder instead of out of the penis. This is called a retrograde ejaculation.

If a man has a retrograde ejaculation, but is still making sperm, it is possible to recover sperm from the urine or bladder. This sperm can be used to fertilize an egg through artificial insemination or in vitro fertilization, which could result in a pregnancy.

Sometimes, the nerves recover from damage due to surgery. It may take several years for this to happen or the nerves may never recover. Nerve sparing techniques are used whenever possible. When surgery involves removal of the prostate or testicles, the ability to ejaculate sperm is affected. Options available for men who lose the ability to have an erection or to ejaculate might include either a penile prosthesis to provide an erection, or sperm banking before surgery for later use in a medically assisted pregnancy. If you have questions about how a surgery may affect your sensations or ability to have children, be sure to discuss this with your doctor before the surgery.

Some cancer surgeries which may alter a man's ability to have an erection or to ejaculate include:

- abdominal perineal resection (APR) (the removal of part of the colon and rectum),

- prostatectomy (the removal of the prostate),

- retroperitoneal lymph node dissection (the removal of lymph nodes from the back of the abdominal cavity),

- radical cystectomy (the removal of the bladder and the prostate),

- orchiectomy (removal of the testicles).

Medically Assisted Ways to Achieve a Pregnancy

The options to start a family have been improved through recent advances in technology. Success is not guaranteed, but it allows men and women the chance to contribute to the genetic make-up of their child.

Sperm Banking

Freezing sperm (cryopreservation), allows men to save or "bank" sperm before undergoing cancer treatment that may reduce or prevent chances of having children. A sample of sperm is collected into a sterile container by masturbation. Two to seven days without sexual activity is advised (prior to the day of collection). This will increase the number of motile (swimming) sperm in the sample. Fewer than two days and greater than seven days can decrease the number of living and swimming sperm in the sample. A small portion of the sample will be thawed, shortly after freezing, to determine the percentage of motile (swimming) sperm that are expected to survive the freezing. On the average, 40% of the sperm are active when thawed. A small sample of the specimen is checked before freezing to determine the quality of the sperm. This information will be important for selecting a technique for future pregnancy attempts.

A semen sample is frozen in a controlled rate freezer which gradually cools the sample to minus 180° Celcius.

Intrauterine Insemination

Intrauterine insemination is a procedure in which the frozen sperm are inserted into the woman's uterus on the day the egg is expected to be released into the fallopian tube. Before insertion the frozen

151

sperm is thawed, washed, and concentrated into a small volume. Along with a quality sperm sample, normal reproductive functions in the woman and skilled timing are required to achieve a pregnancy. This procedure can be performed in a gynecologist's office and is the least expensive medically assisted reproductive technique. The charges for the procedure are usually less than a thousand dollars. The amount covered by insurance varies.

Donor Sperm

Artificial insemination using anonymous donor sperm is a parenting option that is available.

Donor Embryo Program

Couples who have been treated with in vitro fertilization often freeze some of their fertilized eggs (embryos). If they find that they cannot use their frozen embryos they may decide to donate them to a couple that cannot have children. Donated embryos will be offered first to couples who have no living children, or both partners have a problem that interferes with having children.

Medical evaluation including sexually transmitted disease testing and genetic screening will be required of donor participants. Recipients are also prepared by counseling, medical history and examination, and blood tests. Many weeks of hormone medications are given to the woman receiving the donor embryo, to prepare the uterus for a pregnancy.

Emotional Support

The decision to attempt a medically assisted reproductive procedure is one that carries a lot of emotion. There are difficult questions that a couple must think about and discuss before they can come to a decision. What is the prognosis of the partner with the diagnosis of cancer? Is the healthy partner prepared or willing to accept the responsibilities of being a single parent if their partner should relapse or die? What effects will this have on the children and their future? These are very tough questions to think about, but are questions that should be discussed. Counseling is a part of the process if you decide to pursue a medically assisted reproductive procedure. You can also discuss any concerns or questions you have with your doctor before making a decision. Some people may feel that they are in a conflict with their religious beliefs if they choose medically assisted reproduction. These feelings need to be explored with your clergy or religious leader and resolved before you make your final decision.

There may be difficult legal and ethical issues to think about before you plan a medically assisted reproductive technique. Couples who have frozen embryos (fertilized eggs) for future use need to discuss what would be done with the embryos if something happened to one of the partners, or if the marriage was ended before they were used. On the same line, if there is frozen sperm, what should happen to the sperm if the man dies? Should the stored embryos or sperm be destroyed? If there are embryos stored and the couple divorce, should one person be awarded custody rights?

These are legally and ethically charged questions that are very difficult to discuss. If it comes at a time when treatment for cancer is a concern, it is sometimes harder to talk about.

Using donated sperm or donated eggs brings with it a different set of concerns. Will it be more comforting to know the donor or is it better not to know? What will the child need to or want to know about the donor? What should family and friends know about the donor that was involved in your child's birth? All questions need to be answered before deciding to participate in medically assisted reproduction.

There are no guarantees with medically assisted reproduction, but it does allow a chance to have a child. It may take several tries to become pregnant and for some couples it may never happen. Couples should be prepared to handle the feelings of disappointment that may come if they are unable to conceive a child, as well as the feelings experienced when a pregnancy is achieved. Following a pregnancy the possibilities of a miscarriage or birth defects are the same as with a "naturally" conceived pregnancy. Being well informed and prepared to make a decision on the options of medically assisted reproduction will allow you to feel that you have some control over the decision to have a child.

Costs

Financial concerns may decide what options you are able to pursue. Health insurance coverage for the diagnosis and treatment of infertility varies from plan to plan. Some insurance providers pay for both diagnosis and treatment, some pay diagnosis only, and some pay nothing for infertility procedures. It is important for patients to write to insurance providers or call and confirm infertility benefits.

Adoption

Adopting a child is always an option for starting a family. Although it does not allow the parents the ability to contribute to the genetic make-up of the child, they may raise the child as their own. The bond between adoptive parents and their children can be as strong as the bond between biological parents and their children, and the relationship can be as fulfilling.

There are two basic ways of locating an adoptive child: 1) agency assisted or 2) through private adoption.

Agency-Assisted Adoption

There are many agencies that assist with adoptions in the United States. Some agencies specialize in out-of-state adoptions, overseas or out-of-the-country adoptions, or adoption of children that are considered "waiting" to be adopted (these children may be minority, physically or emotionally challenged, older, or part of a group of brothers or sisters).

Agencies may vary in their charges for services or the requirements they have for adoptive parents and birth mothers. Many agencies take time to do pre-adoption screenings of adoptive parents, complete home studies, and check on medical condition and history. For the birth mothers, some agencies ask for health screening for substance abuse and medical fitness. They provide extensive counseling on their decision to place their child up for adoption, health screening, prenatal education, and assistance with pre-natal concerns. When using an agency the process of waiting and preparing for adoption may be very long, and some find it frustrating.

Private Adoption

Private adoption is common and often times a lot faster. Adoptive parents are able to find the birth mother on their own without waiting for an agency. It is a good idea to seek the help of an adoption consultant or an attorney knowledgeable in adoption counseling that can assist you in finding and working with the prospective birth mother. They also provide legal guidance on state laws, rights of the birth parents and legal procedures to close the adoption. Choosing an attorney or consultant carefully is important if you are planning to go with a private adoption. You need to be aware of the laws in your state on adoption so that the proper procedures can be followed to assure closure to the adoption.

Cost of Adoption

The costs to adopt may range in the thousands of dollars. Some factors that affect cost include: private or agency-assisted adoption; in-state, out-of-state, or out-of-country adoption; how much the adoptive parents (legally) are allowed to contribute to the birth mother's pre-natal expenses; and whether an insurance plan covers some of the adoption related costs.

Emotional Support

The process involved with finding an adoptive child can be long and frustrating. There are many legal issues that need to be discussed and it can be hard to understand the process. It can put a strain on all the people involved. Many states have waiting periods where the birth mother or father can change their mind and not allow the child to be adopted. This could occur close to the adoption time or after the child has been placed in their adopted home.

The amount of involvement with the birth parents is something else you may consider. Open adoptions are becoming more accepted and this allows the adoptive parents to meet, or learn something about the birth parents. Some birth parents want to keep ongoing contact with the child after they are adopted. This is something to discuss before adoption and determine what you would be comfortable with.

It may be helpful to seek counseling before getting involved with the adoption process to assist with some of the emotional strains involved with adoption. Often times you can get counseling through the agency or consultant that you may choose to work with.

Conclusion

Wherever you are personally with the decision to start a family, we hope that this chapter has provided you with some helpful information and answered some of the questions that were important to you.

Part Four

Non-Malignant Prostate Conditions and Related Concerns

Chapter 21

Prostatic Enlargement: Benign Prostatic Hyperplasia

The Prostate Gland

The prostate is a walnut-sized gland that forms part of the male reproductive system. The gland is made of two lobes, or regions, enclosed by an outer layer of tissue. As Figure 21.1 shows, the prostate is located in front of the rectum and just below the bladder, where urine is stored. The prostate also surrounds the urethra, the canal through which urine passes out of the body.

Scientists do not know all the prostate's functions. One of its main roles, though, is to squeeze fluid into the urethra as sperm move through during sexual climax. This fluid, which helps make up semen, energizes the sperm and makes the vaginal canal less acidic.

Benign Prostatic Hyperplasia (BPH): A Common Part of Aging

It is common for the prostate gland to become enlarged as a man ages. Doctors call the condition benign prostatic hyperplasia (BPH), or benign prostatic hypertrophy.

As a man matures, the prostate goes through two main periods of growth. The first occurs early in puberty, when the prostate doubles in size. At around age 25, the gland begins to grow again. This second growth phase often results, years later, in BPH.

National Institute of Diabetes and Digestive and Kidney Diseases (NIDDK), NIH Publication Number 98-3012, 2000.

Though the prostate continues to grow during most of a man's life, the enlargement doesn't usually cause problems until late in life. BPH rarely causes symptoms before age 40, but more than half of men in their sixties and as many as 90 percent in their seventies and eighties have some symptoms of BPH.

As the prostate enlarges, the layer of tissue surrounding it stops it from expanding, causing the gland to press against the urethra like a clamp on a garden hose. The bladder wall becomes thicker and irritable. The bladder begins to contract even when it contains small amounts of urine, causing more frequent urination. Eventually, the bladder weakens and loses the ability to empty itself. Urine remains in the bladder. The narrowing of the urethra and partial emptying of the bladder cause many of the problems associated with BPH.

Many people feel uncomfortable talking about the prostate, since the gland plays a role in both sex and urination. Still, prostate enlargement is as common a part of aging as gray hair. As life expectancy rises,

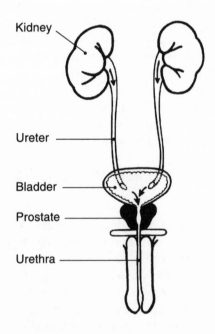

Figure 21.1. Normal urine flow.

so does the occurrence of BPH. In the United States alone, 375,000 hospital stays each year involve a diagnosis of BPH.

It is not clear whether certain groups face a greater risk of getting BPH. Studies done over the years suggest that BPH occurs more often among married men than single men and is more common in the United States and Europe than in other parts of the world. However, these findings have been debated, and no definite information on risk factors exists.

Why BPH Occurs

The cause of BPH is not well understood. For centuries, it has been known that BPH occurs mainly in older men and that it doesn't develop in men whose testes were removed before puberty. For this reason, some researchers believe that factors related to aging and the testes may spur the development of BPH.

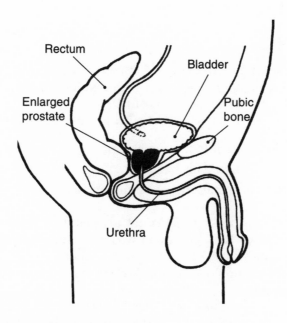

Figure 21.2. *Urine flow with BPH.*

161

Throughout their lives, men produce both testosterone, an important male hormone, and small amounts of estrogen, a female hormone. As men age, the amount of active testosterone in the blood decreases, leaving a higher proportion of estrogen. Studies done with animals have suggested that BPH may occur because the higher amount of estrogen within the gland increases the activity of substances that promote cell growth.

Another theory focuses on dihydrotes-tosterone (DHT), a substance derived from testosterone in the prostate, which may help control its growth. Most animals lose their ability to produce DHT as they age. However, some research has indicated that even with a drop in the blood's testosterone level, older men continue to produce and accumulate high levels of DHT in the prostate. This accumulation of DHT may encourage the growth of cells. Scientists have also noted that men who do not produce DHT do not develop BPH.

Some researchers suggest that BPH may develop as a result of "instructions" given to cells early in life. According to this theory, BPH occurs because cells in one section of the gland follow these instructions and "reawaken" later in life. These "reawakened" cells then deliver signals to other cells in the gland, instructing them to grow or making them more sensitive to hormones that influence growth.

Symptoms

Many symptoms of BPH stem from obstruction of the urethra and gradual loss of bladder function, which results in incomplete emptying of the bladder. The symptoms of BPH vary, but the most common ones involve changes or problems with urination, such as:

- A hesitant, interrupted, weak stream.
- Urgency and leaking or dribbling.
- More frequent urination, especially at night.

The size of the prostate does not always determine how severe the obstruction or the symptoms will be. Some men with greatly enlarged glands have little obstruction and few symptoms while others, whose glands are less enlarged, have more blockage and greater problems.

Sometimes a man may not know he has any obstruction until he suddenly finds himself unable to urinate at all. This condition, called acute urinary retention, may be triggered by taking over-the-counter cold or allergy medicines. Such medicines contain a decongestant drug, known as a sympathomimetic. A potential side effect of this drug may be to prevent the bladder opening from relaxing and allowing urine to empty. When partial obstruction is present, urinary retention also can be brought on by alcohol, cold temperatures, or a long period of immobility.

It is important to tell your doctor about urinary problems such as those described above. In 8 out of 10 cases, these symptoms suggest BPH, but they also can signal other, more serious conditions that require prompt treatment. These conditions, including prostate cancer, can be ruled out only by a doctor's exam.

Severe BPH can cause serious problems over time. Urine retention and strain on the bladder can lead to urinary tract infections, bladder or kidney damage, bladder stones, and incontinence. If the bladder is permanently damaged, treatment for BPH may be ineffective. When BPH is found in its earlier stages, there is a lower risk of developing such complications.

Diagnosis

You may first notice symptoms of BPH yourself, or your doctor may find that your prostate is enlarged during a routine checkup. When BPH is suspected, you may be referred to a urologist, a doctor who specializes in problems of the urinary tract and the male reproductive system. Several tests help the doctor identify the problem and decide whether surgery is needed. The tests vary from patient to patient, but the following are the most common.

Digital Rectal Exam (DRE)

This exam is usually the first test done. The doctor inserts a gloved finger into the rectum and feels the part of the prostate next to the rectum. This exam gives the doctor a general idea of the size and condition of the gland.

Prostate Specific Antigen (PSA) Blood Test

In order to rule out cancer as a cause of urinary symptoms, your doctor may recommend a PSA blood test. PSA, a protein produced by prostate cells, is frequently present at elevated levels in the blood of men who have prostate cancer. The U.S. Food and Drug Administration has approved a PSA test for use in conjunction with a digital rectal exam to help detect prostate cancer in men age 50 or older and for monitoring prostate cancer patients after treatment. However, much remains unknown about the interpretation of PSA levels, the test's ability to discriminate cancer from benign prostate conditions, and the best course of action following a finding of elevated PSA.

Because many unanswered questions surround the issue of PSA screening, the relative magnitude of its potential risks and benefits is unknown. Both PSA and ultrasound tests enhance detection when added to DRE screening. But they are known to have relatively high false-positive rates, and they may identify a greater number of medically insignificant tumors. Thus, PSA screening might lead to treatment of unproven benefit that could result in morbidity (including impotence and incontinence) and mortality. It cannot be determined from earlier studies whether PSA screening will reduce prostate cancer mortality. Ongoing studies are addressing this issue.

Rectal Ultrasound

If there is a suspicion of prostate cancer, your doctor may recommend a test with rectal ultrasound. In this procedure, a probe inserted in the rectum directs sound waves at the prostate. The echo patterns of the sound waves form an image of the prostate gland on a display screen.

Urine Flow Study

Sometimes the doctor will ask a patient to urinate into a special device which measures how quickly the urine is flowing. A reduced flow often suggests BPH.

Intravenous Pyelogram (IVP)

IVP is an x-ray of the urinary tract. In this test, a dye is injected into a vein, and the x-ray is taken. The dye makes the urine visible on the x-ray and shows any obstruction or blockage in the urinary tract.

Cystoscopy

In this exam, the doctor inserts a small tube through the opening of the urethra in the penis. This procedure is done after a solution numbs the inside of the penis so all sensation is lost. The tube, called a cystoscope, contains a lens and a light system, which help the doctor see the inside of the urethra and the bladder. This test allows the doctor to determine the size of the gland and identify the location and degree of the obstruction.

Treatment

Men who have BPH with symptoms usually need some kind of treatment at some time. However, a number of recent studies have questioned the need for early treatment when the gland is just mildly enlarged. These studies report that early treatment may not be needed because the symptoms of BPH clear up without treatment in as many as one-third of all mild cases. Instead of immediate treatment, they suggest regular checkups to watch for early problems. If the condition begins to pose a danger to the patient's health or causes a major inconvenience to him, treatment is usually recommended.

Since BPH may cause urinary tract infections, a doctor will usually clear up any infection with antibiotics before treating the BPH itself. Although the need for treatment is not usually urgent, doctors generally advise going ahead with treatment once the problems become bothersome or present a health risk.

Drug Treatment

Over the years, researchers have tried to find a way to shrink or at least stop the growth of the prostate without using surgery. Recently, several new medications have been tested in clinical trials, and the Food and Drug Administration (FDA) has approved four drugs to treat BPH. These drugs may relieve common symptoms associated with an enlarged prostate.

Finasteride (marketed under the name Proscar), FDA-approved in 1992, inhibits production of the hormone DHT, which is involved with prostate enlargement. Its use can actually shrink the prostate in some men.

FDA also approved the drugs terazosin (marketed as Hytrin) in 1993, doxazosin (marketed as Cardura) in 1995, and tamsulosin (marketed as Flomax) in 1997 for the treatment of BPH. All three drugs act by relaxing the smooth muscle of the prostate and bladder neck to improve urine flow and to reduce bladder outlet obstruction. Terazosin, doxazosin, and tamsulosin belong to the class of drugs known as alpha blockers. Terazosin and doxazosin were developed first to treat high blood pressure. Tamsulosin is the first alpha blocker developed specifically to treat BPH.

Nonsurgical Treatment

Because drug treatment is not effective in all cases, researchers in recent years have developed a number of procedures that relieve BPH symptoms but are less invasive than surgery.

Transurethral Microwave Procedures. In May 1996, FDA approved the Prostatron, a device that uses microwaves to heat and destroy excess prostate tissue. In the procedure called transurethral microwave thermotherapy (TUMT), the Prostatron sends computer-regulated microwaves through a catheter to heat selected portions of the prostate to at least 111 degrees Fahrenheit. A cooling system protects the urinary tract during the procedure.

A similar microwave device, the Targis System, received FDA approval in September 1997. Like the Prostatron, the Targis System delivers microwaves to destroy selected portions of the prostate and uses a cooling system to protect the urethra. A heat-sensing device inserted in the rectum helps monitor the therapy.

Both procedures take about 1 hour and can be performed on an outpatient basis without general anesthesia. Neither procedure has been reported to lead to impotence or incontinence.

While microwave therapy does not cure BPH, it reduces urinary frequency, urgency, straining, and intermittent flow. It does not correct the problem of incomplete emptying of the bladder. Ongoing research will determine any long-term effects of microwave therapy and who might benefit most from this therapy.

Transurethral Needle Ablation. In October 1996, FDA approved Vidamed's minimally invasive Transurethral Needle Ablation (TUNA) System for the treatment of BPH.

The TUNA System delivers low-level radiofrequency energy through twin needles to burn away a well-defined region of the enlarged prostate. Shields protect the urethra from heat damage. The TUNA System improves urine flow and relieves symptoms with fewer side effects when compared with transurethral resection of the prostate (TURP). No incontinence or impotence has been observed.

Surgical Treatment

Most doctors recommend removal of the enlarged part of the prostate as the best long-term solution for patients with BPH. With surgery for BPH, only the enlarged tissue that is pressing against the urethra is removed; the rest of the inside tissue and the outside capsule are left intact. Surgery usually relieves the obstruction and incomplete emptying caused by BPH. The following section describes the types of surgery that are used.

Transurethral Surgery. In this type of surgery, no external incision is needed. After giving anesthesia, the surgeon reaches the prostate by inserting an instrument through the urethra.

A procedure called TURP (transurethral resection of the prostate) is used for 90 percent of all prostate surgeries done for BPH. With TURP, an instrument called a resectoscope is inserted through the penis. The resectoscope, which is about 12 inches long and 1/2 inch in diameter, contains a light, valves for controlling irrigating fluid, and an electrical loop that cuts tissue and seals blood vessels.

During the 90-minute operation, the surgeon uses the resectoscope's wire loop to remove the obstructing tissue one piece at a time. The pieces of tissue are carried by the fluid into the bladder and then flushed out at the end of the operation.

Most doctors suggest using TURP whenever possible. Transurethral procedures are less traumatic than open forms of surgery and require a shorter recovery period.

Another surgical procedure is called transurethral incision of the prostate (TUIP). Instead of removing tissue, as with TURP, this procedure widens the urethra by making a few small cuts in the bladder neck, where the urethra joins the bladder, and in the prostate gland itself. Although some people believe that TUIP gives the same relief as TURP with less risk of side effects such as retrograde ejaculation, its advantages and long-term side effects have not been clearly established.

Open Surgery. In the few cases when a transurethral procedure cannot be used, open surgery, which requires an external incision, may be used. Open surgery is often done when the gland is greatly enlarged, when there are complicating factors, or when the bladder has been damaged and needs to be repaired. The location of the enlargement within the gland and the patient's general health help the surgeon decide which of the three open procedures to use.

With all the open procedures, anesthesia is given and an incision is made. Once the surgeon reaches the prostate capsule, he scoops out the enlarged tissue from inside the gland.

Laser Surgery. In March 1996, FDA approved a surgical procedure that employs side-firing laser fibers and Nd: YAG lasers to vaporize obstructing prostate tissue. The doctor passes the laser fiber through the urethra into the prostate using a cystoscope and then delivers several bursts of energy lasting 30 to 60 seconds. The laser energy destroys prostate tissue and causes shrinkage. Like TURP, laser surgery requires anesthesia and a hospital stay. One advantage of laser surgery over TURP is that laser surgery causes little blood loss. Laser surgery also allows for a quicker recovery time. But laser surgery may not be effective on larger prostates. The long-term effectiveness of laser surgery is not known.

Your Recovery after Surgery in the Hospital

If you have surgery, you'll probably stay in the hospital from 3 to 10 days depending on the type of surgery you had and how quickly you recover.

At the end of surgery, a special catheter is inserted through the opening of the penis to drain urine from the bladder into a collection bag. Called a Foley catheter, this device has a water-filled balloon on the end that is placed in the bladder, which keeps it in place.

This catheter is usually left in place for several days. Sometimes, the catheter causes recurring painful bladder spasms the day after surgery. These may be difficult to control, but they will eventually disappear.

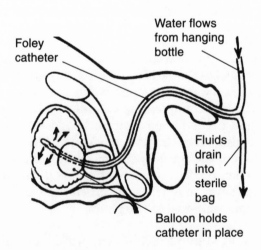

Figure 21.3. Foley Catheter.

168

You may also be given antibiotics while you are in the hospital. Many doctors start giving this medicine before or soon after surgery to prevent infection. However, some recent studies suggest that antibiotics may not be needed in every case, and your doctor may prefer to wait until an infection is present to give them.

After surgery, you will probably notice some blood or clots in your urine as the wound starts to heal. If your bladder is being irrigated (flushed with water), you may notice that your urine becomes red once the irrigation is stopped. Some bleeding is normal, and it should clear up by the time you leave the hospital. During your recovery, it is important to drink a lot of water (up to 8 cups a day) to help flush out the bladder and speed healing.

Do's and Don'ts

Take it easy the first few weeks after you get home. You may not have any pain, but you still have an incision that is healing—even with transurethral surgery, where the incision can't be seen. Since many people try to do too much at the beginning and then have a setback, it is a good idea to talk to your doctor before resuming your normal routine. During this initial period of recovery at home, avoid any straining or sudden movements that could tear the incision. Here are some guidelines:

- Continue drinking a lot of water to flush the bladder.
- Avoid straining when moving your bowel.
- Eat a balanced diet to prevent constipation. If constipation occurs, ask your doctor if you can take a laxative.
- Don't do any heavy lifting.
- Don't drive or operate machinery.

Getting Back to Normal

Even though you should feel much better by the time you leave the hospital, it will probably take a couple of months for you to heal completely. During the recovery period, the following are some common problems that can occur:

- *Problems Urinating.* You may notice that your urinary stream is stronger right after surgery, but it may take awhile before you can urinate completely normally again. After the catheter is removed, urine will pass over the surgical wound on the prostate, and you may initially have some discomfort or feel a sense of urgency when you urinate. This problem will gradually lessen, though, and after a couple of months you should be able to urinate less frequently and more easily.

- *Inability to Control Urination (Incontinence).* As the bladder returns to normal, you may have some temporary problems controlling urination, but long-term incontinence rarely occurs. Doctors find that the longer problems existed before surgery, the longer it will take for the bladder to regain its full function after the operation.

- *Bleeding.* In the first few weeks after transurethral surgery, the scab inside the bladder may loosen, and blood may suddenly appear in the urine. Although this can be alarming, the bleeding usually stops with a short period of resting in bed and drinking fluids. However, if your urine is so red that it is difficult to see through or if it contains clots or if you feel any discomfort, be sure to contact your doctor.

Sexual Function after Surgery

Many men worry about whether surgery for BPH will affect their ability to enjoy sex. Some sources state that sexual function is rarely affected, while others claim that it can cause problems in up to 30 percent of all cases. However, most doctors say that even though it takes awhile for sexual function to return fully, with time, most men are able to enjoy sex again.

Complete recovery of sexual function may take up to 1 year, lagging behind a person's general recovery. The exact length of time depends on how long after symptoms appeared that BPH surgery was done and on the type of surgery. Following is a summary of how surgery is likely to affect the following aspects of sexual function.

Erections

Most doctors agree that if you were potent (able to maintain an erection) shortly before surgery, you will probably be able to have erections afterward. Surgery rarely causes a loss of potency. However, surgery cannot usually restore potency that was lost before the operation.

170

Ejaculation

Although most men are able to continue having erections after surgery, a prostatectomy frequently makes them sterile (unable to father children) by causing a condition called "retrograde ejaculation" or "dry climax."

During sexual activity, sperm from the testes enters the urethra near the opening of the bladder. Normally, a muscle blocks off the entrance to the bladder, and the semen is expelled through the penis. However, the coring action of prostate surgery cuts this muscle as it widens the neck of the bladder. Following surgery, the semen takes the path of least resistance and enters the wider opening to the bladder rather than being expelled through the penis. Later it is harmlessly flushed out with urine.

Orgasm

Most men find little or no difference in the sensation of orgasm, or sexual climax, before and after surgery. Although it may take some time to get used to retrograde ejaculation, you should eventually find sex as pleasurable after surgery as before.

Many people have found that concerns about sexual function can interfere with sex as much as the operation itself. Understanding the surgical procedure and talking over any worries with the doctor before surgery often help men regain sexual function earlier. Many men also find it helpful to talk to a counselor during the adjustment period after surgery.

Is Further Treatment Needed?

In the years after your surgery, it is important to continue having a rectal exam once a year and to have any symptoms checked by your doctor.

Since surgery for BPH leaves behind a good part of the gland, it is still possible for prostate problems, including BPH, to develop again. However, surgery usually offers relief from BPH for at least 15 years. Only 10 percent of the men who have surgery for BPH eventually need a second operation for enlargement. Usually these are men who had the first surgery at an early age.

Sometimes, scar tissue resulting from surgery requires treatment in the year after surgery. Rarely, the opening of the bladder becomes scarred and shrinks, causing obstruction. This problem may require a surgical procedure similar to transurethral incision. More often, scar tissue may form in the urethra and cause narrowing. This problem can usually be solved during an office visit when the doctor stretches the urethra.

Prostatic Stents

Stents are small devices inserted through the urethra to the narrowed area and allowed to expand, like a spring. The stent pushes back the prostatic tissue, widening the urethra. FDA approved the Urolume Endoprosthesis in 1996 to relieve urinary obstruction in men and improve ability to urinate. The device is approved for use in men for whom other standard surgical procedures to correct urinary obstruction have failed.

BPH and Prostate Cancer: No Apparent Relation

Although some of the signs of BPH and prostate cancer are the same, having BPH does not seem to increase the chances of getting prostate cancer. Nevertheless, a man who has BPH may have undetected prostate cancer at the same time or may develop prostate cancer in the future. For this reason, the National Cancer Institute and the American Cancer Society recommend that all men over 40 have a rectal exam once a year to screen for prostate cancer.

After BPH surgery, the tissue removed is routinely checked for hidden cancer cells. In about 1 out of 10 cases, some cancer tissue is found, but often it is limited to a few cells of a nonaggressive type of cancer, and no treatment is needed.

Research in BPH

The National Institute of Diabetes and Digestive and Kidney Diseases (NIDDK) was established by Congress in 1950 as one of the National Institutes of Health (NIH), whose mission is to improve human health through biomedical research. NIH is the research branch of the U.S. Department of Health and Human Services.

NIDDK conducts and supports a variety of research in diseases of the kidney and urinary tract. Much of the research targets disorders of the lower urinary tract, including BPH, urinary tract infection, interstitial cystitis, urinary obstruction, prostatitis, and urinary stones. The knowledge gained from these studies is advancing scientific understanding of why BPH develops and may lead to improved methods of diagnosing and treating prostate enlargement. One such study is the Medical Therapy of Prostatic Symptoms Trial.

Chapter 22

Prostatitis

Prostatitis may account for up to 25 percent of all office visits by young and middle-age men for complaints involving the genital and urinary systems. The term prostatitis actually encompasses four disorders.

Acute Bacterial Prostatitis

Acute bacterial prostatitis is the least common of the four types but also the easiest to diagnose and treat effectively. Men with this disease often have chills, fever, pain in the lower back and genital area, urinary frequency and urgency often at night, burning or painful urination, body aches, and a demonstrable infection of the urinary tract, as evidenced by white blood cells and bacteria in the urine. It is treated with an appropriate antibiotic.

Chronic Bacterial Prostatitis

Chronic bacterial prostatitis is also relatively uncommon. It is acute prostatitis associated with an underlying defect in the prostate, a focal point for bacterial persistence in the urinary tract. Effective treatment usually requires identifying and removing the defect and then treating the infection with antibiotics. However, antibiotics often do not cure it.

National Institute of Diabetes and Digestive and Kidney Diseases (NIDDK); NIH Pub. No. 00-4553, 1999.

Chronic Prostatitis/Chronic Pelvic Pain Syndrome

Chronic prostatitis/chronic pelvic pain syndrome is the most common but least understood form of the disease. It is found in men of any age; symptoms go away and then return without warning. Chronic prostatitis/chronic pelvic pain syndrome may be inflammatory or noninflammatory. In the inflammatory form, urine, semen, and other fluids from the prostate show no evidence of a known infecting organism but do contain cells the body usually produces to fight infection. In the noninflammatory form, no evidence of inflammation, including infection-fighting cells, is present.

Asymptomatic Inflammatory Prostatitis

Asymptomatic inflammatory prostatitis is the diagnosis when the patient does not complain of pain or discomfort but has infection-fighting cells in his semen. Doctors usually find this form of prostatitis when looking for causes of infertility or testing for prostate cancer.

Chapter 23

Impotence

Impotence is a consistent inability to sustain an erection sufficient for sexual intercourse. Medical professionals often use the term "erectile dysfunction" to describe this disorder and to differentiate it from other problems that interfere with sexual intercourse, such as lack of sexual desire and problems with ejaculation and orgasm. This chapter focuses on impotence defined as erectile dysfunction.

Impotence can be a total inability to achieve erection, an inconsistent ability to do so, or a tendency to sustain only brief erections. These variations make defining impotence and estimating its incidence difficult. Experts believe impotence affects between 10 and 15 million American men. In 1985, the National Ambulatory Medical Care Survey counted 525,000 doctor-office visits for erectile dysfunction.

Impotence usually has a physical cause, such as disease, injury, or drug side-effects. Any disorder that impairs blood flow in the penis has the potential to cause impotence. Incidence rises with age: about 5 percent of men at the age of 40 and between 15 and 25 percent of men at the age of 65 experience impotence. Yet, it is not an inevitable part of aging.

Impotence is treatable in all age groups, and awareness of this fact has been growing. More men have been seeking help and returning to near-normal sexual activity because of improved, successful treatments for impotence. Urologists, who specialize in problems of the

National Institute of Diabetes and Digestive and Kidney Diseases (NIDDK); NIH Publication Number 97-3923, 1998.

urinary tract, have traditionally treated impotence—especially complications of impotence.

How Does an Erection Occur?

The penis contains two chambers, called the corpora cavernosa, which run the length of the organ (see Figure 23.1). A spongy tissue fills the chambers. The corpora cavernosa are surrounded by a membrane, called the tunica albuginea. The spongy tissue contains smooth muscles, fibrous tissues, spaces, veins, and arteries. The urethra, which is the channel for urine and ejaculate, runs along the underside of the corpora cavernosa.

Erection begins with sensory and mental stimulation. Impulses from the brain and local nerves cause the muscles of the corpora cavernosa to relax, allowing blood to flow in and fill the open spaces.

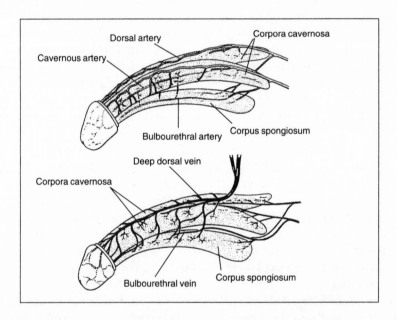

Figure 23.1. *Arteries (top) and veins (bottom) penetrate the long, filled cavities running the length of the penis—the corpora cavernosa and the corpus spongiosum. Erection occurs when relaxed muscles allow the corpora cavernosa to fill with excess blood fed by the arteries, while drainage of blood through the veins is blocked.*

The blood creates pressure in the corpora cavernosa, making the penis expand. The tunica albuginea helps to trap the blood in the corpora cavernosa, thereby sustaining erection. Erection is reversed when muscles in the penis contract, stopping the inflow of blood and opening outflow channels.

What Causes Impotence?

Since an erection requires a sequence of events, impotence can occur when any of the events is disrupted. The sequence includes nerve impulses in the brain, spinal column, and area of the penis, and response in muscles, fibrous tissues, veins, and arteries in and near the corpora cavernosa.

Damage to arteries, smooth muscles, and fibrous tissues, often as a result of disease, is the most common cause of impotence. Diseases—including diabetes, kidney disease, chronic alcoholism, multiple sclerosis, atherosclerosis, and vascular disease—account for about 70 percent of cases of impotence. Between 35 and 50 percent of men with diabetes experience impotence.

Surgery (for example, prostate surgery) can injure nerves and arteries near the penis, causing impotence. Injury to the penis, spinal cord, prostate, bladder, and pelvis can lead to impotence by harming nerves, smooth muscles, arteries, and fibrous tissues of the corpora cavernosa.

Also, many common medicines produce impotence as a side effect. These include high blood pressure drugs, antihistamines, antidepressants, tranquilizers, appetite suppressants, and cimetidine (an ulcer drug).

Experts believe that psychological factors cause 10 to 20 percent of cases of impotence. These factors include stress, anxiety, guilt, depression, low self-esteem, and fear of sexual failure. Such factors are broadly associated with more than 80 percent of cases of impotence, usually as secondary reactions to underlying physical causes.

Other possible causes of impotence are smoking, which affects blood flow in veins and arteries, and hormonal abnormalities, such as insufficient testosterone.

How Is Impotence Diagnosed?

Patient History

Medical and sexual histories help define the degree and nature of impotence. A medical history can disclose diseases that lead to impotence.

A simple recounting of sexual activity might distinguish between problems with erection, ejaculation, orgasm, or sexual desire.

A history of using certain prescription drugs or illegal drugs can suggest a chemical cause. Drug effects account for 25 percent of cases of impotence. Cutting back on or substituting certain medications often can alleviate the problem.

Physical Examination

A physical examination can give clues for systemic problems. For example, if the penis does not respond as expected to certain touching, a problem in the nervous system may be a cause. Abnormal secondary sex characteristics, such as hair pattern, can point to hormonal problems, which would mean the endocrine system is involved. A circulatory problem might be indicated by, for example, an aneurysm in the abdomen. And unusual characteristics of the penis itself could suggest the root of the impotence—for example, bending of the penis during erection could be the result of Peyronie's disease.

Laboratory Tests

Several laboratory tests can help diagnose impotence. Tests for systemic diseases include blood counts, urinalysis, lipid profile, and measurements of creatinine and liver enzymes. For cases of low sexual desire, measurement of testosterone in the blood can yield information about problems with the endocrine system.

Other Tests

Monitoring erections that occur during sleep (nocturnal penile tumescence) can help rule out certain psychological causes of impotence. Healthy men have involuntary erections during sleep. If nocturnal erections do not occur, then the cause of impotence is likely to be physical rather than psychological. Tests of nocturnal erections are not completely reliable, however. Scientists have not standardized such tests and have not determined when they should be applied for best results.

Psychosocial Examination

A psychosocial examination, using an interview and questionnaire, reveals psychological factors. The man's sexual partner also may be interviewed to determine expectations and perceptions encountered during sexual intercourse.

How Is Impotence Treated?

Most physicians suggest that treatments for impotence proceed along a path moving from least invasive to most invasive. This means cutting back on any harmful drugs is considered first. Psychotherapy and behavior modifications are considered next, followed by vacuum devices, oral drugs, locally injected drugs, and surgically implanted devices (and, in rare cases, surgery involving veins or arteries).

Psychotherapy

Experts often treat psychologically based impotence using techniques that decrease anxiety associated with intercourse. The patient's partner can help apply the techniques, which include gradual development of intimacy and stimulation. Such techniques also can help relieve anxiety when physical impotence is being treated.

Drug Therapy

Drugs for treating impotence can be taken orally, injected directly into the penis, or inserted into the urethra at the tip of the penis. In March 1998, the Food and Drug Administration approved sildenafil citrate (marketed as Viagra), the first oral pill to treat impotence. Taken 1 hour before sexual activity, sildenafil works by enhancing the effects of nitric oxide, a chemical that relaxes smooth muscles in the penis during sexual stimulation, allowing increased blood flow. While sildenafil improves the response to sexual stimulation, it does not trigger an automatic erection as injection drugs do. The recommended dos is 50 mg, and the physician may adjust this dose to 100 mg or 25 mg, depending on the needs of the patient. The drug should not be used more than once a day.

Oral testosterone can reduce impotence in some men with low levels of natural testosterone. Patients also have claimed effectiveness of other oral drugs—including yohimbine hydrochloride, dopamine and serotonin agonists, and trazodone—but no scientific studies have proved the effectiveness of these drugs in relieving impotence. Some observed improvements following their use may be examples of the placebo effect, that is, a change that results simply from the patient's believing that an improvement will occur.

Many men gain potency by injecting drugs into the penis, causing it to become engorged with blood. Drugs such as papaverine hydrochloride, phentolamine, and alprostadil (marked as Caverject) widen blood vessels. These drugs may create unwanted side effects, however, including persistent erection (known as priapism) and scarring. Nitroglycerin, a muscle relaxant, sometimes can enhance erection when rubbed on the surface of the penis.

A system for inserting a pellet of alprostadil into the urethra is marketed as MUSE. The system uses a pre-filled applicator to deliver the pellet about an inch deep into the urethra at the tip of the penis. An erection will begin within 8 to 10 minutes and may last 30 to 60 minutes. The most common side effects of the preparation are aching in the penis, testicles, and area between the penis and rectum; warmth or burning sensation in the urethra; redness of the penis due to increased blood flow; and minor urethral bleeding or spotting.

Research on drugs for treating impotence is expanding rapidly. Patients should ask their doctors about the latest advances.

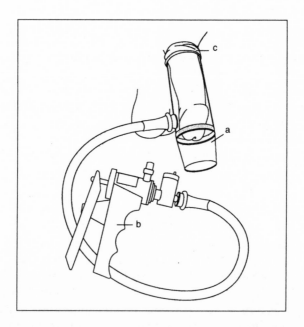

Figure 23.2. *A vacuum-constrictor device causes an erection by creating a partial vacuum around the penis, which draws blood into the corpora cavernosa. Pictured here are the necessary components: (a) a plastic cylinder, which covers the penis; (b) a pump, which draws air out of the cylinder; and (c) an elastic ring, which when fitted over the base of the penis, traps the blood and sustains the erection after the cylinder is removed.*

Vacuum Devices

Mechanical vacuum devices cause erection by creating a partial vacuum around the penis, which draws blood into the penis, engorging it and expanding it. The devices have three components: a plastic cylinder, in which the penis is placed; a pump, which draws air out of the cylinder; and an elastic band, which is placed around the base of the penis, to maintain the erection after the cylinder is removed and during intercourse by preventing blood from flowing back into the body (see Figure 23.2).

One variation of the vacuum device involves a semirigid rubber sheath that is placed on the penis and remains there after attaining erection and during intercourse.

Surgery

Surgery usually has one of three goals:

1. to implant a device that can cause the penis to become erect;
2. to reconstruct arteries to increase flow of blood to the penis;
3. to block off veins that allow blood to leak from the penile tissues.

Implanted devices, known as prostheses, can restore erection in many men with impotence. Possible problems with implants include mechanical breakdown and infection. Mechanical problems have diminished in recent years because of technological advances.

Malleable implants usually consist of paired rods, which are inserted surgically into the corpora cavernosa, the twin chambers running the length of the penis. The user manually adjusts the position of the penis and, therefore, the rods. Adjustment does not affect the width or length of the penis.

Inflatable implants consist of paired cylinders, which are surgically inserted inside the penis and can be expanded using pressurized fluid (see Figure 23.3). Tubes connect the cylinders to a fluid reservoir and pump, which also are surgically implanted. The patient inflates the cylinders by pressing on the small pump, located under the skin in the scrotum. Inflatable implants can expand the length and width of the penis somewhat. They also leave the penis in a more natural state when not inflated.

Surgery to repair arteries can reduce impotence caused by obstructions that block the flow of blood to the penis. The best candidates for such surgery are young men with discrete blockage of an artery because of an injury to the crotch area or fracture of the pelvis. The procedure is less successful in older men with widespread blockage.

Surgery to veins that allow blood to leave the penis usually involves an opposite procedure—intentional blockage. Blocking off veins (ligation) can reduce the leakage of blood that diminishes rigidity of the penis during erection. However, experts have raised questions about this procedure's long-term effectiveness.

What Will the Future Bring?

Advances in suppositories, injectable medications, implants, and vacuum devices have expanded the options for men seeking treatment for impotence. These advances also have helped increase the number of men seeking treatment.

An oral form of the drug phentolamine may soon join sildenafil in the armamentarium of noninvasive treatments for impotence. Other

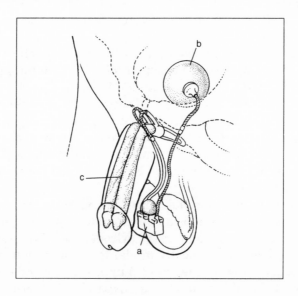

Figure 23.3. With an inflatable implant, erection is produced by squeezing a small pump (a) implanted in the scrotum. The pump causes fluid to flow from a reservoir (b) residing in the lower pelvis to two cylinders (c) residing in the penis. The cylinders expand to create the erection.

treatments in the experimental stages include reconstruction surgery for damaged veins and arteries in the penis. Whether or not this method proves to be safe and effective, ongoing improvements in traditional methods should continue to create more successful and widespread treatment of impotence.

Points to Remember

- Impotence is a consistent inability to sustain an erection sufficient for sexual intercourse.

- Impotence affects 10 to 15 million American men.

- Impotence usually has a physical cause.

- Impotence is treatable in all age groups.

- Treatments include psychotherapy, drug therapy, vacuum devices, and surgery.

Chapter 24

Peyronie's Disease

Peyronie's disease, a condition of uncertain cause, is characterized by a plaque, or hard lump, that forms on the penis. The plaque develops on the upper or lower side of the penis in layers containing erectile tissue. It begins as a localized inflammation and can develop into a hardened scar.

Peyronie's disease often occurs in a mild form that heals without treatment in 6 to 15 months. But in severe cases, the hardened plaque reduces flexibility, causing pain and forcing the penis to bend or arc during erection.

The plaque itself is benign, or noncancerous. A plaque on the top of the shaft (most common) causes the penis to bend upward; a plaque on the underside causes it to bend downward. In some cases, the plaque develops on both top and bottom, leading to indentation and shortening of the penis. At times, pain, bending, and emotional distress prohibit sexual intercourse.

One study found Peyronie's disease occurring in 1 percent of men. Although the disease occurs mostly in middle-aged men, younger and older men can acquire it. About 30 percent of people with Peyronie's disease develop fibrosis (hardened cells) in other elastic tissues of the body, such as on the hand or foot. A common example is a condition known as Dupuytren's contracture of the hand. In some cases, men who are related by blood tend to develop Peyronie's disease, which

National Institute of Diabetes and Digestive and Kidney Diseases (NIDDK); NIH Pub. No. 95-3902, 1998.

suggests that familial factors might make a man vulnerable to the disease.

Men with Peyronie's disease usually seek medical attention because of painful erections and difficulty with intercourse. Since the cause of the disease and its development are not well understood, doctors treat the disease empirically; that is, they prescribe and continue methods that seem to help. The goal of therapy is to keep the Peyronie's patient sexually active. Providing education about the disease and its course often is all that is required. No strong evidence shows that any treatment other than surgery is effective. Experts usually recommend surgery only in long-term cases in which the disease is stabilized and the deformity prevents intercourse.

A French surgeon, François de la Peyronie, first described Peyronie's disease in 1743. The problem was noted in print as early as 1687. Early writers classified it as a form of impotence. Peyronie's disease can be associated with impotence; however, experts now recognize impotence as one factor associated with the disease—a factor that is not always present.

Course of the Disease

Many researchers believe the plaque of Peyronie's disease develops following trauma (hitting or bending) that causes localized bleeding inside the penis. A chamber (actually two chambers known as the corpora cavernosa) runs the length of the penis. The inner-surface membrane of the chamber is a sheath of elastic fibers. A connecting tissue, called a septum, runs along the center of the chamber and attaches at the top and bottom.

If the penis is abnormally bumped or bent, an area where the septum attaches to the elastic fibers may stretch beyond a limit, injuring the lining of the erectile chamber and, for example, rupturing small blood vessels. As a result of aging, diminished elasticity near the point of attachment of the septum might increase the chances of injury.

The damaged area might heal slowly or abnormally for two reasons: repeated trauma and a minimal amount of blood-flow in the sheath-like fibers. In cases that heal within about a year, the plaque does not advance beyond an initial inflammatory phase. In cases that persist for years, the plaque undergoes fibrosis, or formation of tough fibrous tissue, and even calcification, or formation of calcium deposits.

While trauma might explain acute cases of Peyronie's disease, it does not explain why most cases develop slowly and with no apparent traumatic event. It also does not explain why some cases disappear quickly, and why similar conditions such as Dupuytren's contracture do not seem to result from severe trauma.

Treatment

Because the plaque of Peyronie's disease often shrinks or disappears without treatment, medical experts suggest waiting 1 to 2 years or longer before attempting to correct it surgically. During that wait, patients often are willing to undergo treatments that have unproven effectiveness.

Some researchers have given men with Peyronie's disease vitamin E orally in small-scale studies and have reported improvements. Yet, no controlled studies have established the effectiveness of vitamin E therapy. Similar inconclusive success has been attributed to oral application of para-aminobenzoate, a substance belonging to the family of B-complex molecules.

Researchers have injected chemical agents such as collagenase, dimethyl sulfoxide, steroids, and calcium channel blockers directly into the plaques. None of these has produced convincing results. Steroids, such as cortisone, have produced unwanted side effects, such as atrophy, or death of healthy tissues. Perhaps the most promising directly injected agent is collagenase, an enzyme that attacks collagen, the major component of Peyronie's plaques.

Radiation therapy, in which high-energy rays are aimed at the plaque, also has been used. Like some of the chemical treatments, radiation appears to reduce pain, yet it has no effect on the plaque itself and can cause unwelcome side effects. Currently, none of the treatments mentioned here has equalled the body's natural ability to eliminate Peyronie's disease. The variety of agents and methods used points to the lack of a proven, effective treatment.

Peyronie's disease has been treated with some success by surgery. The two most common surgical methods are: removal or expansion of the plaque followed by placement of a patch of skin or artificial material, and removal or pinching of tissue from the side of the penis opposite the plaque, which cancels out the bending effect. The first method can involve partial loss of erectile function, especially rigidity. The second method, known as the Nesbit procedure, causes a shortening of the erect penis.

Some men choose to receive an implanted device that increases rigidity of the penis. In some cases, an implant alone will straighten the penis adequately. In other cases, implantation is combined with a technique of incisions and grafting or plication (pinching or folding the skin) if the implant alone does not straighten the penis.

Most types of surgery produce positive results. But because complications can occur, and because many of the phenomena associated with Peyronie's disease (for example, shortening of the penis) are not corrected by surgery, most doctors prefer to perform surgery only on the small number of men with curvature so severe that it prevents sexual intercourse.

Part Five

Current Research Initiatives and Clinical Trials

Chapter 25

The Prostate Cancer Outcomes Study

The Prostate Cancer Outcomes Study (PCOS) was initiated in 1994 by researchers at the National Cancer Institute (NCI) to look at the impact that treatments for primary prostate cancer have on the quality of life of patients. PCOS is collaborating with six cancer registries that are part of NCI's Surveillance, Epidemiology, and End Results (SEER) Program. (The SEER Program was established by NCI in 1973 to collect cancer data on a routine basis from designated population-based cancer registries in various areas of the country.)

PCOS is the first systematic evaluation of health-related quality-of-life issues for prostate cancer patients conducted on a multiregional scale. It is expected that better knowledge of the effects of treatment will help patients, families, and clinicians make more informed choices about treatment alternatives. PCOS will also provide some of the most detailed data collected on the patterns of prostate cancer care.*

Background

Prostate cancer is the single most common form of non-skin cancer in men in the United States. In the year 2000, an estimated 180,400 men will be diagnosed with prostate cancer, and some 31,900 will die of the disease. Prostate cancer exacts a particularly high toll on African-American men; mortality rates in African-American men are more than twice as high as rates in white men.

Cancer Trials, National Cancer Institute (NCI), 2000.

191

One of the problems facing prostate cancer patients is the uncertainty of many issues surrounding the management of the disease. It is not known, for instance, if the potential benefits of prostate cancer screening outweigh the risks, if surgery is better than radiation, or if treatment is better than no treatment in some cases.

Decisions about treatments are not easy to make. One is that it is difficult for a physician to predict whether a tumor will grow slowly with no health to the patient or will grow quickly and life-threatening. Also, there are no randomized trials that compare the relative benefits of treating early stage patients with radiation therapy, radical prostatectomy (surgical removal of the entire prostate gland along with nearby tissues), or watchful waiting following the patient closely and postponing aggressive therapy unless symptoms of the disease progress). About 80 percent of men diagnosed with prostate cancer have early stage disease.

In spite of all these uncertainties, it is known that certain treatments—radiation therapy, radical prostatectomy, or hormonal therapies—can have detrimental effects on urinary, bowel, and sexual functions. By collecting comprehensive data on the health outcomes of various treatments for prostate cancer, the PCOS will help patients, their families, and physicians make decisions about treatment options.

Patient Population

The Prostate Cancer Outcomes Study uses an already existing population from the NCI SEER tumor registry system. About 3,500 men from six NCI SEER cancer registries including Connecticut, Utah, Mexico, and the metropolitan areas of Atlanta, Ga., Los Angeles, Calif., and Seattle, Wash. are participating in the study. All of the men were diagnosed with primary invasive prostate cancer from Oct. 1, 1994 though Oct. 31, 1995; their tumors were biopsied.

Eighty-eight percent of the patients were diagnosed with clinically localized disease; 4 percent had evidence of cancer in other organs. Forty-two percent of the men were treated with radical prostatectomy, 24 percent with radiotherapy, 13 percent with hormonal therapy, and 22 percent were not treated.

One of the unique features of this study is that the participants represent a large community-based group of patients treated in all types of health care settings, with a substantial number of minority men. In contrast, most previous studies looking at treatment outcomes were limited to a small number of similar men treated in large cancer centers or academic institutions.

Data Collection

A survey questionnaire was sent to patients at six, 12, 24, and 60 months after the initial diagnosis. The survey was designed to focus on quality-of-life issues—urinary, sexual, and bowel dysfunctions—known to be the most relevant to men with prostate cancer. A unique aspect of the PCOS data collection was the extensive effort made to obtain information from medical records of the patients not routinely collected by SEER. These included specific diagnostic procedures, prostate-specific antigen (PSA) values, clinical stage and grade of tumor, details of treatments including specific hormonal therapies, and acute complications of therapies.

Table 25.1. Prostate Cancer Statistics

Estimated new cases, 2000	180,400
Estimated deaths, 2000	31,900
Median age for developing disease	71

Results/Publications

Using the medical records and surveys of the prostate cancer patients, the following PCOS analyses have been published:

Men with clinically localized prostate cancer who are treated with radical prostatectomy are more likely to experience urinary and sexual dysfunction than those treated with external beam radiation therapy. Bowel dysfunction, on the other hand, is more common among men receiving external radiation therapy.

Of the 1,591 men ages 55 to 74 who were treated for localized prostate cancer and followed for two years, those receiving radical prostatectomy (1,156) reported more urinary incontinence (9.6 percent vs. 3.5 percent), and were more bothered by incontinence (11.2 percent vs. 2.3 percent) than men receiving radiotherapy (435). More men treated with prostatectomy also reported being impotent (79.6 percent vs. 62.5 percent), and among men ages 55 to 59 years, the prostatectomy patients were more bothered by their loss of sexual function than were the radiotherapy patients (59.4 percent vs. 25.3 percent). In general, men in the radical prostatectomy group recovered some urinary and sexual function during the second year after treatment, while men in the radiotherapy group remained the same or became slightly worse.

Two years after treatment, men receiving radiotherapy reported more diarrhea (37.2 percent vs. 20.9 percent) and bowel urgency (35.7 percent vs. 14.5 percent) than did men receiving radical prostatectomy. In general, prostatectomy had very little effect on bowel function while radiotherapy patients experienced a decline in bowel function within the first four months of receiving treatment and recovered some function over the two years.

No clear difference in emotional and mental health or overall physical health status was seen between the two groups.

Three factors were found to be the best predictors of the spread of the disease outside the prostate: PSA levels, Gleason score, and age.

The authors were looking for clinical information that could predict spread of prostate cancer outside the capsule that encases the prostate gland (extracapsular extension**) in men who were diagnosed with localized prostate cancer (by biopsy) and treated by radical prostatectomy; 1,395 men participated in this study. The researchers found that the strongest predictors of metastasis were high level of PSA, high Gleason score***, and age greater than 70. They reported that men older than 70 with PSAs greater than 20ng/ml and a Gleason score of eight to 10, had an 85 percent chance of having cancer outside the prostate gland. In contrast, men younger than 50 with PSAs less than 4ng/ml, and a Gleason score less than seven, had a 24 percent chance of having cancer outside the prostate gland. PSA was the strongest single predictor. Ethnicity and region of birth were not useful for predicting metastases. Because nearly half of the men with clinically localized disease undergoing radical prostatectomy had extracapsular extension, many patients may be subjected to the risks and complications of surgery without having a realistic possibility of cure. They also pointed out that physicians may need to reconsider the widely held view that Gleason score is the most important clinical indicator of prognosis.

Radical prostatectomy results in significant sexual dysfunction and some decline in urinary function.

At 18 months or more after surgery, at least 8.4 percent of the patients were incontinent (lost urinary control) and at least 59.9 percent were impotent (unable to achieve an erection sufficient for sexual intercourse). At 24 months, 8.7 percent of men were bothered by the lack of urinary control; 41.9 percent reported that sexual function was a moderate-to-big problem. However, most men were satisfied with their treatment choice.

A small percentage of newly diagnosed prostate cancer cases show evidence of metastases with imaging techniques—bones scans, computerized tomography (CT), and magnetic resonance imaging (MRI).

Less than 5 percent of the imaging studies done for newly diagnosed prostate cancer patients showed evidence of metastases. Specifically, less than 5 percent of men with PSAs between four and 20 showed positive bone scans and less than 2 percent of men with Gleason scores of six or less had positive scans. However, for men with serum PSA levels greater than 50ng/ml and Gleason scores ranging from eight to 10, the imaging studies were positive in over 60 percent of the cases. Reports show that physicians order bone scans on approximately two-thirds of all new patients and CT exams on about one-third of new patients. The low positive yields led the authors to question the cost-effectiveness of ordering imaging among the majority of men with newly diagnosed prostate cancer.

Table 25.2. Trends: Death rates

Black men
> After 1993, lower by 2.3 percent per year on average.

White men
> After 1994, lower by 4.6 percent per year on average.

On-Going Studies

Several on-going analyses are looking at:

- Health outcomes and quality of life following radiation therapy by age and race and type of radiation therapy.

- The effects of different hormonal therapies on sexual function and general quality of life.

- Factors associated with racial/ethnic differences in diagnosis of advanced stage prostate cancer.

- Factors associated with the use of different initial therapies for clinically localized prostate cancer.

- Treatments used for sexual dysfunction after therapy for localized disease.

References

Potosky, A.L., Legler, J., Albertsen, P.C., Stanford, J.L., Gilliland, F.D., Hamilton, A.S., et al., Health outcomes after radical prostatectomy or radiotherapy for clinically localized prostate cancer: Results from the Prostate Cancer Outcomes Study (PCOS). *J Natl Cancer Inst 2000*;92:1582-1592.

Gilliland, F.D., Hoffman, R.M., Hamilton, A., et al., Predicting extracapsular extension of prostate cancer in men treated with radical prostatectomy: results from the population based prostate cancer outcomes study. *J Urology 1999*;162:1341-1345.

Stanford, J.L., Ziding, F., Hamilton, A.S., et al., Urinary and sexual function after radical prostatectomy for clinically localized prostate cancer. *JAMA 2000*;283:354-360.

Albertsen, P.C., Hanley, J.A., Harlan, L.C., Gilliland, F.D., Hamilton, A., Liff, J.M., Stanford, J.L., Stephenson, R.A. The positive yield of imaging studies in the evaluation of men with newly diagnosed prostate cancer: a population based analysis. *J Urology 2000*;163:1138-1143.

Notes

* A more detailed description of PCOS is available in the following publication: Potosky, A.L., Harlan, L.C., Stanford, J.L., et al. Prostate

Cancer Practice Patterns and Quality of Life: the Prostate Cancer Outcomes Study. *J Natl Cancer Inst 1999*;91:1719-1724.

** Extracapsular extension is defined as stage T3 or T4 tumor, positive regional lymph nodes, and tumor at the margin of the excised tumor or metastatses.

*** The Gleason score is a method of grading the degree of differentiation of a tumor. If a cancer is poorly differentiated (looks like an immature cell), it is likely to be more aggressive; a well differentiated cell looks more similar to a normal cell and is usually less aggressive. The Gleason for each reading can range from one to five, with one the most well differentiated and five the most poorly differentiated. A pathologist will look at the two most poorly differentiated parts of the tumor and grade them. The Gleason score is the sum of the two grades, and so can range from two to 10. The higher the score, the poorer the prognosis.

Chapter 26

The Prostate, Lung, Colorectal and Ovarian (PLCO) Cancer Screening Trial

The Prostate, Lung, Colorectal, and Ovarian Cancer Screening Trial, or PLCO Trial, is a large-scale study to determine if certain tests will reduce the number of deaths from these cancers. Sponsored by the National Cancer Institute (NCI), the United States Government's lead agency for cancer research, the study will involve 148,000 men and women ages 55 through 74 at medical facilities in 10 geographic areas across the United States.

Following are a series of questions and answers about the PLCO Cancer Screening Trial, which will be helpful to individuals seeking information about this study.

What is a clinical trial?

A clinical trial is a research study conducted with people. There are many types of clinical trials. They range from studies to prevent, detect, diagnose, and treat a disease, to studies of the psychological impact of the disease and ways to improve a participant's comfort and quality of life.

What is a screening test?

A screening test is a type of examination, done by a health professional, that may find cancer before it causes symptoms or pain. Most people who are tested will not have cancer.

Excerpted from "Q & A about the PLCO Cancer Screening Trial," National Cancer Institute (NCI), 2000.

Why are screening tests for these cancers being studied?

Together, prostate, lung, colorectal, and ovarian cancers account for nearly half of all cancers diagnosed as well as cancer deaths in the United States each year. The tests being studied may detect these cancers before symptoms develop, but whether treatment at this stage will reduce the chance of dying from the diseases is unknown.

Doesn't early detection of cancer offer a better chance for effective treatment and survival?

Some medical experts believe that the earlier prostate, lung, colorectal, and ovarian cancers are detected, the better the chance that treatment will extend or save lives. However, early detection does not necessarily mean that a patient's life is extended. The PLCO Trial is designed to help answer this question.

What screening tests are being studied?

Different tests are being studied for each type of cancer.

- For prostate cancer, men will have a digital rectal exam and a blood test for prostate-specific antigen (known as PSA).

- For lung cancer, men and women will receive a regular chest x-ray.

- For colorectal cancer, men and women will be screened with a lighted instrument called a flexible sigmoidoscope that lets health professionals see inside the rectum and the lower part of the colon.

- For ovarian cancer, women will have a physical exam of the ovaries, a blood test for the tumor marker known as CA-125, and an ultrasound test called transvaginal ultrasound.

Who is eligible to participate in the PLCO Trial?

Doctors expect to enroll 148,000 men and women between the ages of 55 and 74 in the trial at 10 medical centers across the country. These volunteers must not have any of the cancers for which they might be screened in the study, although a diagnosis of other cancers may not exclude their participation.

Men participating in the Prostate Cancer Prevention Trial, who are taking either the drug finasteride (Proscar) or a placebo to assess the drug's effect on the prevention of prostate cancer, are not eligible to participate in the PLCO Trial. Men taking finasteride for any reason are not eligible for the PLCO Trial.

Women participating in the Breast Cancer Prevention Trial, who are at increased risk of breast cancer and are taking either tamoxifen (Nolvadex) or a placebo to assess the drug's ability to prevent the disease, are not eligible to participate in the PLCO Trial.

Why are individuals ages 55 through 74 the only people eligible for this study?

Cancer occurs more often as people grow older. Most cancers (79 percent) occur in people who are age 55 and older. Because risk for the disease is greater in older persons, they are the most appropriate population to study.

Will every participant have every test?

No. The men and women who participate in the PLCO Trial will be randomized (selected by chance) to have either the tests being studied (intervention group) or undergo the usual health care their doctors provide (control group).

Why do only half of the study participants receive the tests being studied?

The benefits of the tests being studied are unknown, and they may not provide any advantage to the participants. By comparing the number of cancers diagnosed and the number of cancer deaths in the intervention and control groups, the researchers will be able to study.

Members of the control group who continue to receive "usual care" from their regular health care providers are not screened at PLCO Trial medical centers, but they will be asked about their personal and family history of cancer and other medical questions. This information is part of the comparison between the groups and will be used to learn more about risks for these diseases. Although they are not having the tests being studied, their participation is vital to the trial.

How much will it cost to participate?

There will be no charge to participants for the screening tests being evaluated. Other medical care costs, such as doctor visits, are not covered because they are part of routine care.

What if cancer is found?

Results of the PLCO Trial tests are sent to the participants and their physicians as soon as they become available. If there are any abnormal test results, the participant will be referred to a physician of his/her choice for diagnostic followup tests. The costs of diagnostic tests and treatments are not covered in the study because they are part of routine medical care.

How often will the tests be conducted?

The intervention group will have the tests at the initial visit and once every year for the next 3 years, except for the sigmoidoscopy exam, which will be performed only twice during the initial visit and during the third year of the trial. The researchers will be in contact with the participants for at least 10 years from the time they enter the study. Participation is voluntary and participants may withdraw from the study at any time.

The researchers will regularly monitor the information received from the participants and the tests conducted. If a benefit from a particular test is seen, that portion of the study may be stopped so that the test can be made available to the general public. Also, if there is a health risk found from administering a test, that part of the study will be modified or stopped.

Do these medical procedures carry some risk?

Even though the potential risks from these tests are minimal, such risks will be fully explained, and information about them is included in a written consent form that each participant signs before enrolling in the trial.

Why is NCI testing digital rectal examination and sigmoidoscopy when the tests are already recommended for screening?

The values of the digital rectal exam in screening for prostate cancer and the sigmoidoscopy exam in screening for colorectal cancer are not well documented. The PLCO Trial will provide vital information on whether use of these exams decreases the number of deaths caused by these cancers.

How can a person enroll in the PLCO Trial?

Men and women who are interested in participating in the PLCO Trial should contact the center nearest to them. Locations of the centers can be obtained by calling the NCI's Cancer Information Service at 1-800-4-CANCER (1-800-422-6237).

Is there information about the trial on the World Wide Web (Internet)?

Information about the PLCO Trial can be found at the following Internet address:

http://dcp.nci.nih.gov/plco

Chapter 27

The Prostate Cancer Prevention Trial (PCPT)

The Trial

The Prostate Cancer Prevention Trial, or PCPT, is a clinical chemoprevention trial designed to see whether taking the drug finasteride (trade name Proscar-R) can prevent prostate cancer in men ages 55 and older. The study, which recruited participants for 3 years beginning in October 1993, is funded by the National Cancer Institute (NCI), the U.S. Government's principal agency for cancer research.

Following are a list of questions and answers about the PCPT which may be helpful to those seeking information about this trial.

What are clinical trials and clinical chemoprevention trials?

Clinical trials are research studies conducted with people. There are many types of clinical trials. They include studies to prevent, detect, diagnose, and treat a disease as well as studies of the psychological impact of the disease and ways to improve a participant's comfort and quality of life.

Chemoprevention trials, one type of clinical trial, look at possible ways to prevent cancer using drugs, vitamins, or other agents. The PCPT is the largest chemoprevention trial ever done with men.

CancerNet, National Cancer Institute (NCI), 2000.

Who is coordinating the PCPT? How long will the trial last?

Researchers with the Southwest Oncology Group (SWOG), based in San Antonio, Texas, are coordinating the study, which is being conducted at 222 sites across the United States. SWOG is a cooperative group of cancer researchers from medical centers around the country. Cooperative groups work with NCI in developing new ways to prevent and treat cancer.

Researchers from two other cooperative groups, the Eastern Cooperative Oncology Group (ECOG) and the Cancer and Leukemia Group B (CALGB), are also participating in the PCPT. The trial is planned to last a total of 10 years. The recruitment for the trial lasted about 3 years, and each man will participate for 7 years.

Who is participating in the PCPT?

Men 55 years of age and older who are in good health and show no evidence of prostate cancer are participating in the study.

Why are only men 55 years of age and older participating in the PCPT?

Many diseases, including prostate cancer, occur more frequently in older persons. The risk of developing prostate cancer increases with age, and about 98 percent of prostate cancer cases occur in men ages 55 and older. Thus, the PCPT's age requirement was set to ensure that men who are at risk for the disease were targeted.

What tests were used to determine eligibility for the PCPT?

To determine their eligibility for the trial, men had a digital rectal exam (DRE) and a blood test for prostate-specific antigen (PSA). These tests are commonly used to help detect prostate cancer. To participate, a man must have had a DRE that showed no sign of prostate cancer, and a PSA blood level of 3.0 ng/ml or less. A PSA of 4.0 ng/ml or less is considered normal, but a cutoff level of 3.0 ng/mg was chosen for the PCPT to reduce the chance that a man may have entered the trial with early, undiagnosed prostate cancer.

Are men with benign prostate enlargement included in the trial?

Men who have an enlarged prostate—a common condition in older men—were included in the trial only if the condition was not severe enough to require immediate treatment. Benign prostate enlargement often causes urinary obstruction, and may be treated with an operation called transurethral resection of the prostate (TURP) or with finasteride or other drugs.

What other factors were considered when enrolling men into the PCPT?

Men who had been diagnosed with any cancer, other than basal cell or squamous cell cancers of the skin were not included in the trial unless they had been free of cancer for at least 5 years. Men who had hormonal therapy (including finasteride or anabolic steroids) or who had chemotherapy or radiation therapy for any cancer, did not meet the eligibility criteria for inclusion into the trial. In addition, men who had urinary retention problems or who were receiving anticoagulant (blood-thinning) medication—excluding aspirin—were not included in the trial.

Will every man in the trial receive finasteride?

The 18,000 men in the PCPT were randomized (selected by chance) to receive either finasteride or a placebo (an inactive pill that looks like finasteride). One-half of the men in the trial take finasteride, and one-half take a placebo. In a process known as "double-blinding," neither the participant nor his physician knows which pill he is receiving. Setting up a trial in this way allows researchers to clearly see what the true benefits and side effects of finasteride may be without the influence of other factors such as the expectations of participants or researchers.

What is the dose of finasteride and how long will it be given?

All men in the trial take one pill per day for up to 7 years, either a 5-milligram dose of finasteride or a placebo.

How much will the finasteride cost?

Participants do not pay for the finasteride or the placebo. The company that manufactures finasteride, Merck and Co., Inc., of Whitehouse Station, New Jersey, is providing both the finasteride and the placebo without charge.

Are men required to have any medical exams?

A blood cholesterol test was done at the time of the first visit to the study site. Participants are required to have annual DREs and PSA blood tests for the duration of the study. If any problem is discovered through a DRE or PSA screening during the course of the study, a prostate biopsy is done at that time to check for prostate cancer. At the end of the 7 years in the trial, each participant will have a biopsy. A prostate biopsy involves removing a small sample of prostate tissue with a needle placed into the prostate gland and examining the sample under a microscope for evidence of cancer.

Who pays for these medical exams?

Annual analysis of blood samples for PSA and the biopsy at the end of 7 years are provided without charge. A cholesterol screening test was provided free of charge to all study participants at the first visit to the study site. The only charge to participants is for routine health care that all men in this age group should have.

Physician, medical examination, and general clinic costs, including DREs and drawing blood for PSA testing, are charged to the participant in the same way as if he were not part of the trial. However, the costs for these tests may be covered by a participant's health insurance. If cancer or other prostate problems are discovered during the regular exams, the participant is referred to his personal physician for appropriate care. Costs for diagnosis and treatment of prostate problems, prostate cancer, or other medical conditions during the 7 years of the study are also the responsibility of the participant.

What are the responsibilities of men participating in this trial?

Men in the PCPT need to be committed to participating in the trial for at least 7 years. They also have to take a pill each day for 7 years, and have to visit the study center every 6 months to pick up a new supply of pills. Men must also have followup examinations (DRE, PSA, and physical exam) once a year. At the time of these exams, they also are required to complete some forms and questionnaires. Participants must also report any side effects they experience. Every effort is made to make followup appointments convenient and to ensure that all men who participate in the trial feel comfortable with their involvement. Although participants may withdraw at any time for any reason, the trial's success will depend on the continued participation of men who enrolled.

Finasteride

What is finasteride?

Finasteride is a drug, taken by mouth as a pill, that is used to treat patients with symptomatic noncancerous enlargement of the prostate, also known as benign prostatic hyperplasia (BPH). The U.S. Food and Drug Administration (FDA) approved the drug for this use in 1992. However, it has never before been used in an attempt to prevent cancer.

How does finasteride work in treating benign prostate enlargement?

Finasteride reduces levels of dihydrotestosterone (DHT), a male hormone that is important in normal and abnormal prostate growth. DHT plays a key role in benign prostate enlargement and is also believed to be involved in the development of prostate cancer.

Finasteride works by blocking the action of an enzyme, 5-alpha reductase, that is needed to convert the hormone testosterone into DHT. Because the chemical structure of finasteride resembles that of testosterone, it binds to 5-alpha reductase, making the enzyme unavailable for the conversion of testosterone to DHT.

Why is finasteride being tested to prevent prostate cancer?

The development of prostate cancer is strongly influenced by male hormones. DHT in particular is known to be important for the growth of prostate cells. Because finasteride reduces levels of DHT, researchers believe the drug may prevent the cellular changes that can lead to prostate cancer. In support of this hypothesis, finasteride has been shown to inhibit the growth of prostate cancer cells in tissue culture ("test tube") experiments. Studies have shown that men with inherited 5-alpha reductase deficiency have not developed prostate cancer.

Can finasteride cause side effects?

Like most medications, whether over-the-counter preparations, prescription drugs, or drugs in clinical trials, finasteride may cause side effects. Finasteride primarily affects the prostate, and its side effects appear to be infrequent and relatively mild—an important consideration when testing a drug in healthy people.

In the manufacturer's clinical trials, carried out to gain FDA approval to market finasteride, approximately 1,100 men with benign prostate enlargement were given either finasteride or a placebo. Side effects were observed in a small number of men in both groups. Decreased sexual desire was reported by 3.3 percent of men given finasteride, compared with 1.6 percent of men given a placebo; impotence (difficulty achieving an erection) was reported by 3.7 percent of the finasteride group, compared with 1.1 percent of the placebo group; and decreased ejaculatory volume was reported by 2.8 percent of the finasteride group, compared with 0.9 percent of the placebo group.

It is unknown how much finasteride can be absorbed by a woman's body through semen, or whether finasteride could harm a developing male fetus. Because of these uncertainties, a man whose sexual partner could become pregnant should discuss this issue thoroughly with the study physician.

Because finasteride is a relatively new drug, the possibility remains that other side effects will be identified after more men have taken it for longer periods of time. Participants in the PCPT are asked twice a year about side effects and are encouraged to call the study site any time they have symptoms or concerns they feel may be related to the trial.

Other Questions

What is the prostate gland?

The prostate is a male sex gland. It produces a thick fluid that forms part of semen, enabling sperm to be released during ejaculation. The normal prostate is about the size of a walnut, and is located below the bladder and in front of the rectum. The prostate surrounds the upper part of the urethra, the tube that empties urine from the bladder.

How common is prostate cancer?

Prostate cancer is the most frequently diagnosed cancer among American men, other than skin cancer. In 2000, about 180,400 men will be diagnosed with prostate cancer in the United States, and about 31,900 men will die of the disease.

Who is at risk of developing or dying of prostate cancer?

Age is the most common risk factor for prostate cancer. The disease is rare in men under age 45, but incidence rates rise rapidly with age. Annual U.S. incidence rates from 1993 to 1997 were 50.8 cases per 100,000 men under age 65, and 1,025.3 cases per 100,000 men ages 65 and older. Most men who get prostate cancer are in their seventies or older.

Men with a family history of prostate cancer are at increased risk for the disease. Black men have higher incidence rates than white men, though incidence among white men is rising faster, probably as a result of intensified screening. Mortality rates among black men are twice as high as those of white men. This may be partly due to the fact that black men, on average, are diagnosed at later stages of disease than white men.

Why is the PCPT so important?

Prostate cancer is an important public health problem. Although the number of men being diagnosed with prostate cancer has decreased slightly in the past few years, 1997 incidence rates (the latest available) are nearly double the incidence rates from 20 years earlier. The decline in heart disease mortality in recent decades means that more men are living to older ages at which risk for prostate cancer is highest.

The hormone dependence of prostate growth offers one possible avenue of intervention before cancer has a chance to develop. Finasteride works in treating benign prostate enlargement by altering the hormonal balance in the prostate. The PCPT is testing whether finasteride may prevent prostate cancer through the same hormonal mechanism. A large, controlled clinical trial is the only way to determine whether the benefits outweigh any risk, and whether finasteride should be approved for general use as a preventive agent. The drug's relatively mild side effects make it a good candidate for testing in healthy people.

The researchers are also using reports of participants to assess the effects of finasteride on men's sexual and urinary functioning and other quality-of-life measures. In addition, the trial gives researchers an opportunity to observe the effect of finasteride on PSA levels of men taking the drug, and to study the usefulness of DRE and PSA as screening tests for prostate cancer.

How will healthy men benefit from participating in the PCPT?

Although finasteride's effectiveness is currently unknown, researchers hope that the drug will prevent prostate cancer from occurring in men receiving it in the trial. All participants receive regular exams. Some men wanted to participate because they are at increased risk for the disease. Men receiving finasteride may experience shrinkage of existing prostate enlargement, although this is not a direct aim of the study. In addition, men may find satisfaction in contributing to medical science and perhaps helping other men who may benefit from the results of the trial in the future.

Chapter 28

Taking Part in Clinical Trials: What to Expect

What Are Clinical Trials?

Why Are Clinical Trials Important?

Clinical trials, also called cancer treatment or research studies, test new treatments in people with cancer. The goal of this research is to find better ways to treat cancer and help cancer patients. Clinical trials test many types of treatment such as new drugs, new approaches to surgery or radiation therapy, new combinations of treatments, or new methods such as gene therapy.

A clinical trial is one of the final stages of a long and careful cancer research process. The search for new treatments begins in the laboratory, where scientists first develop and test new ideas.

If an approach seems promising, the next step may be testing a treatment in animals to see how it affects cancer in a living being and whether it has harmful effects. Of course, treatments that work well in the lab or in animals do not always work well in people. Studies are done with cancer patients to find out whether promising treatments are safe and effective.

Clinical trials are important in two ways. First, cancer affects us all, whether we have it, care about someone who does, or worry about getting it in the future. Clinical trials contribute to knowledge and progress against cancer. If a new treatment proves effective in a study, it may become a new standard treatment that can help many patients.

National Cancer Institute (NCI), NIH Publication Number 97-4250, 1998.

Many of today's most effective standard treatments are based on previous study results. Examples include treatments for breast, colon, rectal, and childhood cancers. Clinical trials may also answer important scientific questions and suggest future research directions. Because of progress made through clinical trials, many people treated for cancer are now living longer.

Second, the patients who take part may be helped personally by the treatment(s) they receive. They get up-to-date care from cancer experts, and they receive either a new treatment being tested or the best available standard treatment for their cancer. Of course, there is no guarantee that a new treatment being tested or a standard treatment will produce good results. New treatments also may have unknown risks. But if a new treatment proves effective or more effective than standard treatment, study patients who receive it may be among the first to benefit. Some patients receive only standard treatment and benefit from it.

In the past, clinical trials were sometimes seen as a last resort for people who had no other treatment choices. Today, patients with common cancers often choose to receive their first treatment in a clinical trial.

What Happens in a Clinical Trial?

In a clinical trial, patients receive treatment and doctors carry out research on how the treatment affects the patients. While clinical trials have risks for the people who take part, each study also takes steps to protect patients.

What Is It Like to Receive Treatment in a Study?

When you take part in a clinical trial, you receive your treatment in a cancer center, hospital, clinic, and/or doctor's office. Doctors, nurses, social workers, and other health professionals may be part of your treatment team. They will follow your progress closely. You may have more tests and doctor visits than you would if you were not taking part in a study. You will follow a treatment plan your doctor prescribes, and you may also have other responsibilities such as keeping a log or filling out forms about your health. Some studies continue to check on patients even after their treatment is over.

How Is the Research Carried Out? How Are Patients Protected?

In clinical trials, both research concerns and patient well-being are important. To help protect patients and produce sound results, research with people is carried out according to strict scientific and ethical principles. These include:

1. Each clinical trial has an action plan (protocol) that explains how it will work.

The study's investigator, usually a doctor, prepares an action plan for the study. Known as a protocol, this plan explains what will be done in the study and why. It outlines how many people will take part in the study, what medical tests they will receive and how often, and the treatment plan. The same protocol is used by each doctor that takes part.

For patient safety, each protocol must be approved by the organization that sponsors the study (such as the National Cancer Institute (NCI)) and the Institutional Review Board (IRB) at each hospital or other study site. This board, which includes consumers, clergy, and health professionals, reviews the protocol to try to be sure that the research will not expose patients to extreme or unethical   risks.

2. Each study enrolls people who are alike in key ways.

Each study's protocol describes the characteristics that all patients in the study must have. Called eligibility criteria, these guidelines differ from study to study, depending on the research purpose. They may include age, gender, the type and stage of cancer, and whether cancer patients who have had prior cancer treatment or who have other health problems can take part.

Using eligibility criteria is an important principle of medical research that helps produce reliable results. During a study, they help protect patient safety, so that people who are likely to be harmed by study drugs or other treatments are not exposed to the risk. After results are in, they also help doctors know which patient groups will benefit if the new treatment being studied is proven to work. For instance, a new treatment may work for one type of cancer but not for another, or it may be more effective for men than women.

3. Cancer clinical trials include research at three different phases.

Each phase answers different questions about the new treatment. Phase I trials are the first step in testing a new treatment in humans. In these studies, researchers look for the best way to give a new treatment (e.g., by mouth, IV drip, or injection? how many times a day?).

They also try to find out if and how the treatment can be given safely (e.g., best dose?); and they watch for any harmful side effects. Because less is known about the possible risks and benefits in Phase I, these studies usually include only a limited number of patients who would not be helped by other known treatments.

Phase II trials focus on learning whether the new treatment has an anticancer effect (e.g., Does it shrink a tumor? improve blood test results?). As in Phase I, only a small number of people take part because of the risks and unknowns involved.

Phase III trials compare the results of people taking the new treatment with results of people taking standard treatment (e.g., Which group has better survival rates? fewer side effects?). In most cases, studies move into Phase III testing only after a treatment shows promise in Phases I and II. Phase III trials may include hundreds of people around the country.

4. In Phase III trials, people are assigned at random to receive either the new treatment or standard treatment.

Researchers assign patients by chance either to a group taking the new treatment (called the treatment group) or to a group taking standard treatment (called the control group). This method, called randomization, helps avoid bias: having the study's results affected by human choices or other factors not related to the treatments being tested.

In some studies, researchers do not tell the patient whether he or she is in the treatment or control group (called a single blind study). This approach is another way to avoid bias, because when people know what drug they are taking, it might change the way they react. For instance, patients who knew they were taking the new treatment might expect it to work better and report hopeful signs because they want to believe they are getting well. This could bias the study by making results look better than they really were.

Why Do Phase III Clinical Trials Compare Treatment Groups?

Comparing similar groups of people taking different treatments for the same type of cancer is another way to make sure that study results are real and caused by the treatment rather than by chance or other factors. Comparing treatments with each other often shows clearly which one is more effective or has fewer side effects.

Another reason Phase III trials compare the new treatment with standard treatment is so that no one in a study is left without any treatment when standard treatment is available, which would be unethical. When no standard treatment exists for a cancer, some studies compare a new treatment with a placebo (a look-alike pill that contains no active drug). However, you will be told if this is a possibility before you decide whether to take part in a study.

Your Doctor Can Tell You More

If you have any questions about how clinical trials work, ask your doctor, nurse, or other health professional. It may be helpful to bring this booklet and discuss points you want to understand better.

Should I Take Part in a Clinical Trial?

This is a question only you, those close to you, and your health professionals can answer together. Learning you have cancer and deciding what to do about it is often overwhelming. This section has information you can use in thinking about your choices and making your decision.

Clinical Trials: Weighing the Pros and Cons

While a clinical trial is a good choice for some people, this treatment option has possible benefits and drawbacks. Here are some factors to consider. You may want to discuss them with your doctor and the people close to you.

Possible Benefits

- Clinical trials offer high-quality cancer care. If you are in a study and do not receive the new treatment being tested, you will receive the best standard treatment. This may be as good as, or better than, the new approach.

- If a new treatment approach is proven to work and you are taking it, you may be among the first to benefit.

- By looking at the pros and cons of clinical trials and your other treatment choices, you are taking an active role in a decision that affects your life.

- You have the chance to help others and improve cancer treatment.

217

Possible Drawbacks

- New treatments under study are not always better than, or even as good as, standard care. They may have side effects that doctors do not expect or that are worse than those of standard treatment.

- Even if a new treatment has benefits, it may not work for you. Even standard treatments, proven effective for many people, do not help everyone.

- If you receive standard treatment instead of the new treatment being tested, it may not be as effective as the new approach.

- Health insurance and managed care providers do not always cover all patient care costs in a study. What they cover varies by plan and by study. To find out in advance what costs are likely to be paid in your case, talk to a doctor, nurse or social worker from the study.

Your Rights, Your Protections

Before and during a cancer treatment study, you have a number of rights. Knowing these can help protect you from harm.

- Taking part in a treatment study is up to you. It may be only one of your treatment choices. Talk with your doctor. Together, you can make the best choice for you.

- If you do enter a study, doctors and nurses will follow your response to treatment carefully throughout the research.

- If researchers learn that a treatment harms you, you will be taken off the study right away. You may then receive other treatment from your own doctor.

- You have the right to leave a study at any time.

One of your key rights is the right to informed consent. Informed consent means that you must be given all the facts about a study before you decide whether to take part. This includes details about the treatments and tests you may receive and the possible benefits and risks they may have. The doctor or nurse will give you an informed consent form that goes over key facts. If you agree to take part in the study, you will be asked to sign this informed consent form.

The informed consent process continues throughout the study. For instance, you will be told of any new findings regarding your clinical trial, such as new risks. You may be asked to sign a new consent form if you want to stay in the study.

Signing a consent form does not mean you must stay in the study. In fact, you can leave at any time. If you choose to leave the study, you will have the chance to discuss other treatments and care with your own doctor or a doctor from the study.

Questions You Should Ask

Finding answers and making choices may be hard for people with cancer and those who care about them. It is important to discuss your treatment choices with your doctor, a cancer specialist (an oncologist) to whom your doctor may refer you, and the staff of any clinical trial you consider entering.

Ask questions about the information you receive during the informed consent process and about any other issues that concern you. Getting answers can help you work better with the doctor. You may want to take a friend or relative along when you talk to the doctor. It also may help to write down your questions and the answers you receive, or bring a tape recorder to record what is said. No question about your care is foolish. It is very important to understand your choices.

Here are some questions you may want to ask about:

The Study

- What is the purpose of the study? In what phase is this study?

- Why do researchers believe the new treatment being tested may be effective? Has it been tested before?

- Who sponsors the study, and who has reviewed and approved it?

- How are the study data and patient safety being checked?

- When and where will study results and information go?

Possible Risks and Benefits

- What are the possible short- and long-term risks, side effects, and benefits to me?

- Are there standard treatments for my type of cancer?

219

- How do the possible risks, side effects, and benefits in the study compare with standard treatment?

Your Care

- What kinds of treatments, medical tests, or procedures will I have during the study? Will they be painful? How do they compare with what I would receive outside the study?

- How often and for how long will I receive the treatment, and how long will I need to remain in the study? Will there be follow-up after the study?

- Where will my treatment take place? Will I have to be in the hospital? If so, how often and for how long?

- How will I know if the treatment is working?

- Will I be able to see my own doctor? Who will be in charge of my care?

Personal Issues

- How could the study affect my daily life?

- Can you put me in touch with other people who are in this study?

- What support is there for me and my family in the community?

Cost Issues

- Will I have to pay for any treatment, tests, or other charges?

- What is my health insurance likely to cover?

- Who can help answer any questions from my insurance company or managed care plan?

Others Can Help

As you make your treatment decisions, remember that you are not alone. Doctors, nurses, social workers, other people with cancer, clergy, family, and those who care about you can help and support you.

Glossary

This glossary contains a list of words used in this chapter and their definitions. It also explains some other terms related to treatment studies that you may hear from your doctor or nurse.

Bias: Human choices or any other factors beside the treatments being tested that affect a study's results. Clinical trials use many methods to avoid bias, because biased results may not be correct.

Clinical trials: Research studies that involve people. Each study tries to answer scientific questions and to find better ways to prevent or treat cancer.

Control group: In a clinical trial, the group of people that receives standard treatment for their cancer.

Informed consent: The process in which a person learns key facts about a clinical trial or research study and then agrees voluntarily to take part or decides against it. This process includes signing a form that describes the benefits and risks that may occur if the person decides to take part.

Institutional Review Board (IRB): Groups of scientists, doctors, clergy, and consumers at each health care facility at which a clinical trial takes place. Designed to protect patients who take part in studies, IRBs review and must approve the protocols for all clinical trials funded by the Federal Government. They check to see that the study is well-designed, does not involve undue risks, and includes safeguards for patients.

Investigator: A researcher in a treatment study.

Oncologist: A doctor who specializes in treating cancer.

Placebo: A tablet, capsule, or injection that looks like the drug or other substance being tested but contains no drug.

Protocol: An action plan for a clinical trial. The plan states what will be done in the study and why. It outlines how many people will take part in the study, what types of patients may take part, what tests they will receive and how often, and the treatment plan.

Randomization: A method used to prevent bias in research. People are assigned by chance to either the treatment or control group.

Remission: When the signs and symptoms of cancer go away, the disease is said to be "in remission." A remission can be temporary or permanent.

Side effects: Problems that occur when treatment affects healthy cells. Common side effects of standard cancer treatments are fatigue, nausea, vomiting, decreased blood cell counts, hair loss, and mouth sores. New treatments being tested may have these or other unknown side effects.

Single blind study: A method used to prevent bias in treatment studies. In a single blind study, the patient is not told whether he/she is taking the standard treatment or the new treatment being tested. Only the doctors know.

Stage: The extent of a cancer and whether the disease has spread from the original site to other parts of the body. Numbers with or without letters are used to define cancer stages (e.g., Stage IIb).

Standard treatment: The best treatment currently known for a cancer, based on results of past research.

Treatment group: The group that receives the new treatment being tested during a study.

Additional Resources

You may want more information for yourself, your family, and your doctor. The following National Cancer Institute (NCI) services are available to help you.

Telephone

Cancer Information Service (CIS)
Toll-free: 800-4-CANCER (800-422-6237)
TTY: 800-332-8615

Provides accurate, up-to-date information on cancer to patients and their families, health professionals, and the general public. Information specialists translate the latest scientific information into understandable language and respond in English, Spanish, or on TTY equipment.

Internet

The following websites may be useful:

http://www.nci.gov
NCI's primary web site contains information about the Institute and its programs.

http://cancertrials.nci.nih.gov

cancerTrials is NCI's comprehensive clinical trials information center for patients, health professionals, and the public. Includes information on understanding trials, deciding whether to participate in trials, finding specific trials, plus research news and other resources.

http://cancernet.nci.nih.gov

CancerNet™ contains material for health professionals, patients, and the public, including information from PDQ(r) about cancer treatment, screening, prevention, supportive care, and clinical trials, and CANCERLIT(r), a bibliographic data base.

E-Mail

CancerMail
cancermail@icicc.nci.nih.gov

Includes NCI information about cancer treatment, screening, prevention, and supportive care. To obtain a contents list, send e-mail to cancermail@icicc.nci.nih.gov with the word "help" in the body of the message.

Publications

Cancer patients, their families and friends, and others may find the following National Cancer Institute books useful. They are available free of charge by calling 1-800-4-CANCER.

"Chemotherapy and You: A Guide to Self-Help During Treatment"

"Eating Hints for Cancer Patients Before, During, and After Treatment"

"Get Relief From Cancer Pain"

"Helping Yourself During Chemotherapy"

"Questions and Answers About Pain Control: A Guide for People with Cancer and Their Families"

"Taking Time: Support for People With Cancer and the People Who Care About Them"

"Taking Part in Clinical Trials: What Cancer Patients Need to Know"

Publications Available in Spanish

"Datos sobre el tratamiento de quimioterapia contra el cancer"

"El tratamiento de radioterapia; guia para el paciente durante el tratamiento"

"En que consisten los estudios clinicos? Un folleto para los pacientes de cancer"

Chapter 29

New Prostate Treatment Technology

Patients with Advanced Prostate Cancer May Benefit from Bone-Targeted Drug

Men with prostate cancer that has spread to the bones may live longer if given a combination of chemotherapy and a bone-targeted radiation drug, according to research reported in the February 3, 2001, issue of the *Lancet*. While most men survive five years or more with early prostate cancer, those diagnosed at later stages don't live nearly as long. In fact, in cases where prostate cancer has spread to the bones and is resistant to standard hormonal therapy, the average life expectancy is nine months.

The phase II clinical trial, reported in the *Lancet*, was designed to test the effectiveness of the combination treatment for patients with advanced disease that was no longer responding to hormone treatments. The study showed gains in survival time and pain relief in men who received chemotherapy treatment plus a drug called strontium-89 (Sr-89). Sr-89 is a radioactive substance used to relieve bone pain caused by metastatic prostate cancer. When injected by vein, Sr-89 moves into bones and works by delivering radiation directly to cancer that has spread there.

The study, led by Shi-Ming Tu, M.D., and colleagues from the University of Texas' M.D. Anderson Cancer Center, involved 103 patients who had advanced prostate cancer that was no longer responsive to

Cancer Trials, National Cancer Institute (NCI), 2001.

hormone therapy. In the first part of the study, all patients received an eight-week course of induction chemotherapy (therapy aimed at shrinking the cancer and determining responsiveness to treatment) using the drugs ketoconazole, doxorubicin, estramustine and vinblastine. After completion of induction chemotherapy, those patients whose prostate cancer was responding (72 patients), went on to enter the second part of the study in which they received consolidation chemotherapy consisting of doxorubicin for six weeks. (Consolidation therapy is treatment given after induction therapy to reduce the number of cancer cells even further.) At this point, patients were also randomly assigned to receive a single dose of Sr-89 or a placebo in addition to the doxorubicin.

On average, the group of 36 patients that received the Sr-89 lived almost a year longer than the group that did not receive it. Of the 103 initial patients in this study, 67 have died. The average survival time for all 103 patients was 18 months. Of the 36 patients who went on to receive consolidation therapy and Sr-89, 22 are still alive and the average survival is 28 months. Of those 36 patients who received consolidation therapy without Sr-89, 27 have died and the average survival time is 17 months.

The study's authors noted that although the results require confirmation, they do strongly support the hypothesis that a bone-targeted consolidation therapy containing Sr-89 improves the clinical outcome of patients with advanced prostate cancer. In previous studies, Sr-89 had not been shown to change the course or prognosis of advanced prostate cancer. In an editorial in the same issue of the *Lancet*, Alexandre Zlotta of the University Clinics of Brussels, Belgium, wrote that the study does not provide definite answers about the beneficial effect of doxorubicin and strontium, but does give researchers strong justification to study more bone-targeted therapies in advanced cases of prostate cancer. While the improvement in survival with Sr-89 was statistically significant, further studies with larger patient populations will be required to compare this promising combination against the hormonal treatment now commonly used for distant metastatic prostate cancer.

Chapter 30

Vitamin E for Prevention of Prostate Cancer

Study in Finland Suggests Vitamin E Prevents Prostate Cancer

The latest analysis from a large prevention trial conducted by the National Cancer Institute (NCI) and the National Public Health Institute of Finland shows that long-term use of a moderate-dose vitamin E supplement substantially reduced prostate cancer incidence and deaths in male smokers. The report was published in the March 18, 1998, issue of the *Journal of the National Cancer Institute*, and the lead author is Olli P. Heinonen, M.D., D.Sc., of the Department of Public Health, University of Helsinki, Finland.

This report from the Alpha-Tocopherol, Beta-Carotene Cancer Prevention Study (ATBC Study) showed that 50- to 69-year-old men who took 50 mg of alpha-tocopherol (a form of the antioxidant vitamin E) daily for 5 to 8 years had 32 percent fewer diagnoses of prostate cancer and 41 percent fewer prostate cancer deaths compared with men who did not receive vitamin E. This dose of vitamin E is equal to about 50 international units (the measure more commonly used with supplements) and is about three times the Recommended Dietary Allowance. The 29,133 male smokers from Finland were randomly assigned to receive alpha-tocopherol, beta-carotene (20 mg), or a placebo (an inactive pill that looked like the vitamin) daily.

"These results give hope that a simple intervention may one day help reduce a man's chances of developing and dying from prostate

Cancer Facts, National Cancer Institute (NCI), 1998.

227

cancer," said Demetrius Albanes, M.D., one of NCI's lead investigators on the study. "But it is important that other studies be done to confirm the beneficial effects of vitamin E. The ATBC Study and similar trials have shown us that supplements are not necessarily magic bullets and, more importantly, that what may be a beneficial supplement for some people may be harmful to others," said Albanes, who is in the Cancer Prevention Studies Branch of NCI's Division of Clinical Sciences.

As an example, he noted that earlier results from the ATBC Study showed that men who took the beta-carotene supplement had 16 percent more cases of lung cancer and 14 percent more lung cancer deaths than those who did not take beta-carotene. Men who drank large amounts of alcohol, and who took the beta-carotene, had higher rates of lung cancer than men who drank less alcohol.

In the current analysis, men taking beta-carotene supplements had more prostate cancer as well, but this increase was not statistically significant and was limited to men who drank alcohol. Men taking both nutrients (beta-carotene and vitamin E) had fewer cases of prostate cancer compared with men on placebo.

In men taking the vitamin E, there was a reduction in clinically detectable prostate cancers beginning within 2 years of starting the supplement—a result which suggests to Philip R. Taylor, M.D., Sc.D., chief of NCI's Cancer Prevention Studies Branch, that vitamin E may be blocking a prostate tumor's progression to a more aggressive state. Most older men have microscopic areas of cancer in their prostate, few of which will progress to life-threatening disease.

"We know that prostate cancer develops first as latent cancer that can't be detected clinically," said Taylor. "For some men, these tumors are transformed from subclinical cancer—which may never affect a man's health—into aggressive disease. We think vitamin E is working by blocking the changeover from these more benign tumors to potentially life-threatening disease."

The investigators do not think that vitamin E affected symptoms that would cause a man to have medical attention, which would lead to a diagnosis of cancer. Overall, men taking vitamin E had fewer diagnoses of later stage cancers than men not taking the supplement. The number of cancers diagnosed at earlier stages, when symptoms are few, was equivalent between supplement and placebo groups.

Prostate-specific antigen (PSA) testing was not common in Finland at the time of the study, and no other screening tests for prostate cancer were done as part of the ATBC Study. Most men diagnosed with prostate cancer had visited their physician with a complaint of urinary difficulties, while others sought medical care for other reasons but mentioned urinary problems, which then were evaluated. Blood samples were taken from the ATBC participants during the study, and using these, an analysis of the value of blood PSA levels in predicting prostate cancer is under way.

In the United States, prostate cancer is the most frequently diagnosed cancer in males, with 184,500 cases expected in 1998 along with 39,200 deaths. African American men have the highest rates of prostate cancer in the United States.

References

Heinonen, O.P., Albanes, D., Virtamo, J., et al. Prostate cancer and supplementation with alpha-tocopherol and beta-carotene: incidence and mortality in a controlled trial. *Journal of the National Cancer Institute* 1998; 90:440-446.

The Alpha-Tocopherol, Beta-Carotene Cancer Prevention Study Group. The effect of vitamin E and beta-carotene on the incidence of lung cancer and other cancers in male smokers. *New England Journal of Medicine* 1994; 330:1029-1035.

Albanes, D., Heinonen, O.P., Taylor, P.R., et al. Alpha-tocopherol and beta-carotene supplements and lung cancer incidence in the alpha-tocopherol, beta-carotene Cancer Prevention Study: effects of baseline characteristics and study compliance. *Journal of the National Cancer Institute* 1996; 88:1560-1570.

Questions and Answers about Prostate Cancer Incidence and Mortality in the Alpha-Tocopherol, Beta-Carotene Cancer Prevention Study

What is the Alpha-Tocopherol, Beta-Carotene Cancer Prevention Study?

The Alpha-Tocopherol, Beta-Carotene Cancer Prevention Study, or ATBC Study, was a chemoprevention trial conducted by the National Cancer Institute (NCI) and the National Public Health Institute of Finland. The purpose of the study was to see if certain vitamin supplements would prevent lung cancer and other cancers in a group of 29,133 male smokers in Finland. The 50- to 69-year-old participants took a pill containing 50 milligrams (mg) alpha-tocopherol (a form of vitamin E), 20 mg beta-carotene (a precursor of vitamin A), both, or a placebo (an inactive pill that looked like the vitamin) daily for 5 to 8 years.

What is a chemoprevention trial?

A chemoprevention trial is a type of clinical trial, which is a research study conducted with people. In a cancer chemoprevention trial, natural or man-made substances are tested to see if they prevent cancer. The people who participate in such a study are healthy or are at risk of developing cancer, or in some studies, people who have been treated for cancer and are at a risk of developing a second cancer.

What were the results of the ATBC Study?

In 1994 and 1996, the ATBC researchers reported that 16 percent more lung cancers were diagnosed and 14 percent more lung cancer deaths occurred in study participants taking beta-carotene. Vitamin E had no effect on lung cancer.

In the new report, ATBC researchers have shown that the participants taking vitamin E had 32 percent fewer cases of prostate cancer and 41 percent fewer deaths from prostate cancer.

Why was the ATBC Study conducted in Finland?

The study was conducted in Finland because of the high lung cancer rates in men in that country, which are due primarily to cigarette smoking. Furthermore, Finland has a clinic system for the screening and treatment of lung diseases (mainly tuberculosis) through which the recruited population of smokers could participate in the study. Finland also has a national cancer registry, which keeps track of all the cancer cases identified in that country, a vital measurement for the large trial.

Why was the trial conducted only in men?

Finnish women were not included in the study because their rate of lung cancer was substantially lower than the rate for Finnish men. In 1985, the annual age-adjusted lung cancer rate for Finnish men was 67 cases per 100,000 men and for women the rate was 8 cases per 100,000 women.

Are the ATBC Study results applicable to Americans?

As a whole, the white men of Finland are similar to white men in the United States, and live similar Western lifestyles. However, in

Finland the population is very uniform, with few ethnic and racial differences, so the relationship of these study results to specific minorities is less clear.

How do prostate cancer rates compare in U.S. men and Finnish men?

Using world standardized rates, the incidence rate of prostate cancer in the United States was 118.6 per 100,000 in 1994, including all races. The U.S. mortality rate was 17.3 per 100,000. In Finland, the 1995 incidence rate was 61.4 per 100,000 and the death rate was 17.9 per 100,000.

Why are prostate cancer incidence rates higher in the United States?

Although there are no clear answers, prostate cancer incidence rates in the United States may be higher in part because of the popularity of prostate-specific antigen (PSA) testing, which identifies cancers that cannot be found by clinical exam. PSA testing for early detection of prostate cancer is generally not done in Finland. Prostate cancer is also a disease of aging and affluence, and historically Finns had a lower life expectancy and standard of living than Americans. Currently, Finns and Americans share very similar lifestyles.

What causes prostate cancer?

The causes of prostate cancer are not yet understood. Age is a factor: most cases are diagnosed in men over age 55 years. Some families have higher incidence of prostate cancer, suggesting inherited susceptibility may influence the development of the disease. Hormones, including testosterone, may play a role. Many other possible factors may be involved, but are not proven or not well understood— men who have had vasectomies, farmers, workers exposed to the metal cadmium, workers in the rubber industry, and smokers may have a greater chance of developing prostate cancer.

Diets high in fat have been suggested to increase risk, while diets high in fruits and vegetables seem to decrease risk. A recent study suggested that supplements of selenium may reduce the risk of prostate cancer.

231

How does the normal Finnish diet compare with the U.S. diet?

he average Finnish diet used to be very high in saturated fat and low in fruits and vegetables. At the time the ATBC Study began, the fat content of the Finnish diet was about 38 percent of total calories. However, the national average fat intake has decreased to about 34 percent of calories from fat, equal to the current U.S. average. The Finns also eat a lot of whole-grain products, like dark rye breads, which gives them a higher fiber intake, and they eat more dairy products. Dietary vitamin E intake is somewhat lower in Finland than in the United States (10 mg versus 17 mg per day).

Why were vitamin E and beta-carotene chosen for this trial?

Vitamin E and beta-carotene were chosen because epidemiologic studies have linked high dietary intake and high serum levels of these micronutrients to a reduced risk of cancer, particularly lung cancer. Both are antioxidants, compounds that may prevent carcinogens from damaging DNA.

How might vitamin E protect against prostate cancer?

The mechanisms by which vitamin E may reduce prostate cancer risk are not clear. Vitamin E is an antioxidant. Antioxidants are compounds that may prevent carcinogens from damaging DNA. In addition to its antioxidant activity, there are a number of possible mechanisms by which vitamin E may be working: vitamin E affects cell membranes, may inhibit the proliferation of cells, may stimulate the immune system or alter sex hormones, and could play a role in inhibiting or increasing apoptosis (programmed cell death). It also plays a role in inducing differentiation (the maturing of cells) and protecting the metabolic pathways that rid the body of toxins.

What doses of these supplements were given in the ATBC Study?

The dose of vitamin E was 50 mg per day of synthetic dl-alpha-tocopheryl acetate, which is equal to 50 international units (IU) of vitamin E. Most multivitamins have about 30 IU of vitamin E, and singular supplements most often have a minimum of 100 IU of vitamin E.

232

The dose of beta-carotene was 20 mg per day of synthetic beta-carotene. The men in the study took one pill each day, which contained vitamin E, beta-carotene, both, or neither.

Did vitamin E have any effect on other causes of death?

Overall, the number of deaths in men taking vitamin E was similar to men not taking vitamin E. The men taking vitamin E were found to have fewer deaths from ischemic heart disease and ischemic stroke (a deficit of blood to the brain due to a constriction of a blood vessel), but more deaths due to all cancers and hemorrhagic stroke (a deficit of blood to the brain due to the rupture of a blood vessel).

What foods are major sources of alpha-tocopherol (vitamin E)?

Vitamin E is found mainly in oils, such as vegetable oils, and in nuts and grains. The amount in the U.S. diet varies, but is estimated to be about 17 mg per day. The top sources of vitamin E in the U.S. diet are salad dressings and mayonnaise; margarine; ready-to-eat cereals; cakes, cookies, and donuts; tomatoes; and eggs.

Should Americans take vitamin E supplements?

NCI has never recommended that Americans take supplements. The results of the ATBC Study, while promising, do not answer whether vitamin E supplements would be able to reduce the risk of prostate cancer in men of varying race and ethnicity and in nonsmokers. There is also concern that men taking vitamin E in this study had more of one type of stroke than men who did not take vitamin E. While the number of men in the ATBC Study who had this type of stroke (hemorrhagic stroke) was small, this possible side effect of vitamin E supplementation needs careful study.

Should Americans avoid taking beta-carotene supplements?

The results from the ATBC Study and the Beta-Carotene and Retinol Efficacy Trial (CARET) suggest that smokers should avoid taking beta-carotene supplements. The best advice for smokers who want to reduce their risk of lung cancer and many other cancers is still the most direct: Stop smoking.

The results of the only large-scale study of beta-carotene in primarily nonsmoking men, the Physicians' Health Study, showed no benefit or harm from taking beta-carotene supplements every other day for 12 years. For all Americans who wish to reduce their risk of cancer, a low-fat diet with plenty of fruits, vegetables, and whole grains remains the choice to make.

How much did the study cost?

NCI allocated about $20 million over 10 years for the trial, with a similar sum contributed by the government and research institutions in Finland. In addition, F. Hoffmann-LaRoche, Ltd., a pharmaceutical company based in Basel, Switzerland, supplied the 60 million pills the men took during the trial, without charge, at a cost to the company of about $3 million.

What other large-scale chemoprevention studies are under way?

NCI has a number of different agents under study, including calcium, fiber, tamoxifen, finasteride, and others. The only ongoing large-scale study of vitamin E is the Women's Health Study, headed by researchers at Boston's Brigham and Women's Hospital.

In the Women's Health Study, which began in 1992, 40,000 healthy women age 50 and older were recruited to take combinations of 50 mg beta-carotene, 600 mg vitamin E, 100 mg aspirin, or placebos every other day. After disappointing results from other beta-carotene trials were announced in January 1996, the beta-carotene portion of the study was dropped. The women are being monitored for cancer and heart disease benefits.

Part Six

Additional Help and Information

Chapter 31

Important Terms for Prostate Patients

A

abdomen (AB-do-men): The part of the body that contains the pancreas, stomach, intestines, liver, gallbladder, and other organs.

adrenal glands (ah-DREE-nal): Two glands located above the kidneys (one above each kidney). They produce several kinds of hormones, including a small amount of sex hormones.

acute (uh-KYOOT): Acute often means urgent. An acute disease happens suddenly. It lasts a short time. Acute is the opposite of chronic, or long lasting.

adjuvant therapy (AD-joo-vant): Treatment given after the primary treatment to make it work better. Adjuvant therapy may include chemotherapy, radiation therapy, or hormone therapy.

albuminuria (AL-byoo-mih-NOO-ree-uh): More than normal amounts of a protein called albumin in the urine. Albuminuria may be a sign of kidney disease.

Excerpted from "What You Need to Know about Cancer," National Cancer Institute, NIH Pub. No. 00-1566, 2000; "What You Need to Know about Prostate Cancer," National Cancer Institute, NIH Pub. No. 96-1576, 1996; and "Urologic Diseases Dictionary," National Institute of Diabetes and Digestive and Kidney Diseases (NIDDK), NIH Pub. No. 00-4376, 1999; and "Prostate Cancer Treatment Options," by David A. Cooke, MD. © 2001 Omnigraphics, Inc.

anesthesia (an-es-THEE-zha): Loss of feeling or awareness. Local anesthetics cause loss of feeling in a part of the body. General anesthetics put the person to sleep.

antiandrogen (an-tee-AN-dro-jen): A drug that blocks the action of male sex hormones.

antidiuretic hormone (ADH) (AN-tee-DY-uh-RET-ik): A natural body chemical that slows down the production of urine.

anuria (uh-NYOO-ree-uh): A condition in which the body stops making urine.

anus (AY-nus): The opening at the lower end of the rectum through which solid waste leaves the body.

B

balloon dilation (dy-LAY-shun): A treatment for benign prostatic hyperplasia or prostate enlargement. A tiny balloon is inflated inside the urethra to make it wider so urine can flow more freely from the bladder.

barium enema: A procedure in which a liquid with barium in it is put into the rectum and colon by way of the anus. Barium is a silver-white metallic compound that helps to show the image of the lower gastrointestinal tract on an x-ray.

benign (beh-NINE): Not cancerous; does not invade nearby tissue or spread to other parts of the body.

benign prostatic hyperplasia (BPH) (prah-STAT-ik HY-per-PLAY-sha): An enlarged prostate not caused by cancer. BPH can cause problems with urination because the prostate squeezes the urethra at the opening of the bladder.

biological therapy (by-o-LAHJ-i-kul): Treatment to stimulate or restore the ability of the immune system to fight infection and disease. Also used to lessen side effects that may be caused by some cancer treatments. Also known as immunotherapy, biotherapy, or biological response modifier (BRM) therapy.

biopsy (BY-ahp-see): A procedure used to remove cells or tissues to look at them under a microscope and check for signs of disease. When an entire tumor or lesion is removed, the procedure is called an excisional biopsy. When only a sample of tissue is removed, the procedure is called an incisional biopsy or core biopsy. When a sample of tissue or fluid is removed with a needle, the procedure is called a needle biopsy or fine-needle aspiration.

bladder (BLAD-ur): The balloon-shaped organ inside the pelvis that holds urine.

bladder control: See continence.

blood urea nitrogen (BUN) (yoo-REE-uh NY-truh-jen): A waste product in the blood that comes from the breakdown of food protein. The kidneys filter blood to remove urea. As kidney function decreases, the BUN level increases.

bone marrow transplantation (trans-plan-TAY-shun): A procedure to replace bone marrow destroyed by treatment with high doses of anticancer drugs or radiation. Transplantation may be autologous (an individual's own marrow saved before treatment), allogeneic (marrow donated by someone else), or syngeneic (marrow donated by an identical twin).

brachytherapy (BRAKE-ih-THER-a-pee): A procedure in which radioactive material sealed in needles, seeds, wires, or catheters is placed directly into or near a tumor. Also called internal radiation, implant radiation, or interstitial radiation therapy.

C

calcium (KAL-see-um): A mineral that the body needs for strong bones and teeth. Calcium may form stones in the kidney.

cancer: A term for diseases in which abnormal cells divide without control. Cancer cells can invade nearby tissues and can spread through the bloodstream and lymphatic system to other parts of the body.

carcinogen (kar-SIN-o-jin): Any substance that causes cancer.

catheter (KATH-uh-ter): A tube that is inserted through the urethra to the bladder to drain urine.

central nervous system (CNS): The brain and spinal cord.

cerebrospinal fluid (CSF) (seh-REE-bro-SPY-nal): The fluid flowing around the brain and spinal cord. Cerebrospinal fluid is produced in the ventricles in the brain.

chemotherapy (kee-mo-THER-a-pee): Treatment with anticancer drugs.

chronic (KRAH-nik): Lasting a long time. Chronic diseases develop slowly. Chronic renal failure may develop over many years and lead to end-stage renal disease.

chronic prostatitis (PRAH-stah-TY-tis): Inflammation of the prostate gland, developing slowly and lasting a long time.

clinical trial: A research study that tests how well new medical treatments or other interventions work in people. Each study is designed to test new methods of screening, prevention, diagnosis, or treatment of a disease.

collagen (KAHL-uh-jen): The major protein found in tissues, cartilage, and bones. Collagen injections are used to treat stress urinary incontinence.

colonoscope (ko-LAHN-o-skope): A thin, lighted tube used to examine the inside of the colon.

colony-stimulating factors: Substances that stimulate the production of blood cells. Colony-stimulating factors include granulocyte colony-stimulating factors (also called G-CSF and filgrastim), granulocyte-macrophage colony-stimulating factors (also called GM-CSF and sargramostim), and promegapoietin.

computed tomography (tuh-MAH-gra-fee): A series of detailed pictures of areas inside the body; the pictures are created by a computer linked to an x-ray machine. Also called computed tomography (CT) scan or computerized axial tomography (CAT) scan.

continence (KON-tih-nents): The ability to control the timing of urination or a bowel movement.

cryosurgery: A procedure that uses extremely cold liquid nitrogen to destroy cancer cells.

cystine stone (SIS-teen): A rare form of kidney stone consisting of the amino acid cystine.

cystinuria (SIS-tih-NOO-ree-uh): A condition in which urine contains high levels of the amino acid cystine. If cystine does not dissolve in the urine, it can build up to form kidney stones.

cystitis (sis-TY-tis): Inflammation of the bladder, causing pain and a burning feeling in the pelvis or urethra.

cystocele (SIS-toh-seel): Fallen bladder. When the bladder falls or sags from its normal position down to the pelvic floor, it can cause either urinary leakage or urinary retention.

cystometrogram (SIS-toh-MET-roh-gram): A line graph that records urinary bladder pressure at various volumes.

cystoscope (SIS-toh-scope): A tube-like instrument used to look inside the bladder.

cystoscopy (sist-OSS-ko-pee): A procedure in which the doctor inserts a lighted instrument through the urethra (the tube leading from the bladder to the outside of the body) to look inside the bladder.

D

digital rectal examination (DRE): An examination in which a doctor inserts a lubricated, gloved finger into the rectum to feel for abnormalities.

dry orgasm: Sexual climax without the release of semen.

dysplasia (dis-PLAY-zha): Cells that look abnormal under a microscope but are not cancer.

E

ejaculation: The release of semen through the penis during orgasm.

endoscopy (en-DAHS-ko-pee): The use of a thin, lighted tube (called an endoscope) to examine the inside of the body.

enuresis (EN-yoo-REE-sis): Urinary incontinence not caused by a physical disorder.

erectile dysfunction (ee-REK-tile dis-FUNK-shun): The inability to get or maintain an erection for satisfactory sexual intercourse. Also called impotence.

erection (ee-REK-shun): Enlargement and hardening of the penis caused by increased blood flow into the penis and decreased blood flow out of it as a result of sexual excitement.

estrogen (ES-tro-jin): A female sex hormone.

excisional biopsy (ek-SI-zhun-al BY-op-see): A surgical procedure in which an entire lump or suspicious area is removed for diagnosis. The tissue is then examined under a microscope.

external radiation (ray-dee-AY-shun): Radiation therapy that uses a machine to aim high-energy rays at the cancer. Also called external-beam radiation.

F

fecal occult blood test (FEE-kul o-KULT): A test to check for blood in stool. (Fecal refers to stool; occult means hidden.)

fertility (fer-TIL-i-tee): The ability to produce children.

five-year survival: This is often used to compare different kinds of treatment for prostate cancer. It is the percentage of patients who can expect to still be alive five years after a given treatment. It is not a "cure" rate; it is simply the odds of surviving five years, with or without cancer.

G

gene: The functional and physical unit of heredity passed from parent to offspring. Genes are pieces of DNA, and most genes contain the information for making a specific protein.

genitals (JEN-ih-tuls): Sex organs, including the penis and testicles in men and the vagina and vulva in women.

genitourinary system (GEN-i-toe-YOO-rin-air-ee): The parts of the body that play a role in reproduction, getting rid of waste products in the form of urine, or both.

Gleason score: A number between two and ten assigned by a pathologist who has examined biopsy specimens from a patient with prostate cancer. This score helps predict how aggressive (likely to spread) the tumor will be. Higher numbers indicate a more dangerous cancer.

grade: How closely a tumor resembles normal tissue of its same type. Suggests the tumor's most likely rate of growth. In prostate cancer, this may be referred to as the Gleason score.

graft-versus-host disease (GVHD): A reaction of donated bone marrow or peripheral stem cells against a person's tissue.

H

hematuria (HEE-muh-TOOR-ee-uh): Blood in the urine, which can be a sign of a kidney stone or other urinary problem.

hormone (HOR-mone): A natural chemical produced in one part of the body and released into the blood to trigger or regulate particular functions of the body. Antidiuretic hormone tells the kidneys to slow down urine production.

hormone therapy: Treatment of cancer by removing, blocking, or adding hormones. Also called endocrine therapy.

hydronephrosis (HY-droh-nef-ROH-sis): Swelling at the top of the ureter, usually because something is blocking the urine from flowing into or out of the bladder.

hypercalciuria (HY-per-kal-see-YOO-ree-uh): Abnormally large amounts of calcium in the urine.

hyperoxaluria (HY-per-ox-uh-LOO-ree-uh): Unusually large amounts of oxalate in the urine, leading to kidney stones.

hypospadias (HY-poh-SPAY-dee-us): A birth defect in which the opening of the urethra, called the urinary meatus, is on the underside of the penis instead of at the tip.

I

imaging: Tests that produce pictures of areas inside the body.

immune system (im-YOON): The body's system for protecting itself from viruses and bacteria or any "foreign" substances.

immunosuppressant (im-YOON-oh-suh-PRESS-unt): A drug given to suppress the natural immune responses. Immunosuppressants are given to transplant patients to prevent organ rejection or to patients with autoimmune diseases like lupus.

immunotherapy (IM-yoo-no-THER-a-pee): Treatment to stimulate or restore the ability of the immune system to fight infection and disease. Also used to lessen side effects that may be caused by some cancer treatments. Also called biological therapy or biological response modifier (BRM) therapy.

impotence (IM-puh-tents): The inability to get or maintain an erection of the penis for sexual activity. Also called erectile dysfunction.

incision (in-SI-zhun): A cut made during surgery.

incisional biopsy (in-SI-zhun-al BY-op-see): A surgical procedure in which a portion of a lump or suspicious area is removed for diagnosis. The tissue is then examined under a microscope.

incontinence (in-KON-tih-nents): Loss of bladder or bowel control; the accidental loss of urine or feces.

infertility: The inability to produce children.

interferon (in-ter-FEER-on): A biological response modifier (a substance that can improve the body's natural response to disease). Interferons interfere with the division of cancer cells and can slow tumor growth. There are several types of interferons, including interferon-alpha, -beta, and -gamma. These substances are normally produced by the body. They are also made in the laboratory for use in treating cancer and other diseases.

interleukin-2 (IL-2) (in-ter-LOO-kin): A type of biological response modifier (a substance that can improve the body's natural response to disease) that stimulates the growth of certain disease-fighting blood cells in the immune system. These substances are normally produced by the body. Aldesleukin is IL-2 that is made in the laboratory for use in treating cancer and other diseases.

internal radiation (ray-dee-AY-shun): A procedure in which radioactive material sealed in needles, seeds, wires, or catheters is placed directly into or near the tumor. Also called brachytherapy, implant radiation, or interstitial radiation therapy.

interstitial cystitis (IC): (IN-ter-STISH-ul sis-TY-tis): A disorder that causes the bladder wall to become swollen and irritated, leading to scarring and stiffening of the bladder, decreased bladder capacity, and, in rare cases, ulcers in the bladder lining. IC is also known as painful bladder syndrome.

intraperitoneal chemotherapy (IN-tra-per-ih-toe-NEE-al KEE-mo-THER-a-pee): Treatment in which anticancer drugs are put directly into the abdominal cavity through a thin tube.

intrathecal chemotherapy (in-tra-THEE-kal KEE-mo-THER-a-pee): Anticancer drugs that are injected into the fluid-filled space between the thin layers of tissue that cover the brain and spinal cord.

Intravenous (IV) (in-tra-VEE-nus): Injected into a blood vessel.

intravenous pyelogram (IN-truh-VEE-nus PY-loh-gram): An x-ray of the urinary tract. A dye is injected to make urine visible on the x-ray and show any blockage in the urinary tract.

K

kidneys (KID-neez): The two bean-shaped organs that filter wastes from the blood. The kidneys are located near the middle of the back. They send urine to the bladder through tubes called ureters.

kidney stone: A stone that develops from crystals that form in urine and build up on the inner surfaces of the kidney, in the renal pelvis, or in the ureters.

L

laparotomy (lap-a-RAH-toe-mee): A surgical incision made in the wall of the abdomen.

leukemia (loo-KEE-mee-a): Cancer of blood-forming tissue.

local therapy: Treatment that affects cells in the tumor and the area close to it.

luteinizing hormone-releasing hormone (LHRH) agonist (LOO-tin-eye-zing AG-o-nist): A substance that closely resembles LHRH, which controls the production of sex hormones. However, LHRH agonists affect the body differently than does LHRH. LHRH agonists keep the testicles from producing hormones.

lymph node: A rounded mass of lymphatic tissue that is surrounded by a capsule of connective tissue. Also known as a lymph gland. Lymph nodes are spread out along lymphatic vessels and contain many lymphocytes, which filter the lymphatic fluid (lymph).

lymphatic system (lim-FAT-ik): The tissues and organs that produce, store, and carry white blood cells that fight infection and other diseases. This system includes the bone marrow, spleen, thymus, and lymph nodes and a network of thin tubes that carry lymph and white blood cells. These tubes branch, like blood vessels, into all the tissues of the body.

lymphoma (lim-FO-ma): Cancer that arises in cells of the lymphatic system.

M

malignant (ma-LIG-nant): Cancerous; a growth with a tendency to invade and destroy nearby tissue and spread to other parts of the body.

medical oncologist (on-KOL-o-jist): A doctor who specializes in diagnosing and treating cancer using chemotherapy, hormonal therapy, and biological therapy. A medical oncologist often serves as the main caretaker of someone who has cancer and coordinates treatment provided by other specialists.

metastasis (meh-TAS-ta-sis): The spread of cancer from one part of the body to another. Tumors formed from cells that have spread are called "secondary tumors" and contain cells that are like those in the original (primary) tumor. The plural is metastases.

monoclonal antibodies (MAH-no-KLO-nul AN-tih-BAH-deez): Laboratory-produced substances that can locate and bind to cancer cells wherever they are in the body. Many monoclonal antibodies are used in cancer detection or therapy; each one recognizes a different protein on certain cancer cells. Monoclonal antibodies can be used alone, or they can be used to deliver drugs, toxins, or radioactive material directly to a tumor.

magnetic resonance imaging (MRI) (mag-NET-ik REZ-o-nans IM-a-jing): A procedure in which a magnet linked to a computer is used to create detailed pictures of areas inside the body.

mutation: Any change in the DNA of a cell. Mutations may be caused by mistakes during cell division, or they may be caused by exposure to DNA-damaging agents in the environment. Mutations can be harmful, beneficial, or have no effect. If they occur in cells that make eggs or sperm, they can be inherited; if mutations occur in other types of

246

cells, they are not inherited. Certain mutations may lead to cancer or other diseases.

N

neoadjuvant therapy: Treatment given before the primary treatment. Neoadjuvant therapy can be chemotherapy, radiation therapy, or hormone therapy.

nephrogenic diabetes insipidus (NEF-roh-JEN-ik DY-uh-BEE-teez in-SIP-ih-dus): Constant thirst and frequent urination because the kidney tubules cannot respond to antidiuretic hormone and therefore pass too much water.

nephrotic syndrome (nef-RAH-tik): A collection of symptoms that indicate kidney damage. Symptoms include high levels of protein in the urine, lack of protein in the blood, and high blood cholesterol.

neurogenic bladder (NEW-roh-JEN-ik): Loss of bladder control caused by damage to the nerves controlling the bladder.

nuclear scan (NEW-klee-ur): A test of the structure, blood flow, and function of the kidneys. The doctor injects a mildly radioactive solution into an arm vein and uses x-rays to monitor its progress through the kidneys.

O

oncologist (on-KOL-o-jist): A doctor who specializes in treating cancer. Some oncologists specialize in a particular type of chance treatment. For example, a radiation oncologist treats cancer with radiation.

orchiectomy (or-kee-EK-to-mee): Surgery to remove the testicles.

overactive bladder: A condition in which the patient experiences two or all three of the following conditions:

urinary urgency
urge incontinence
urinary frequency—defined for this condition as urination more than seven times a day or more than twice at night.

oxalate (AHK-suh-late): A chemical that combines with calcium in urine to form the most common type of kidney stone (calcium oxalate stone).

P

painful bladder syndrome: Another name for interstitial cystitis.

pathologist (pa-THOL-o-jist): A doctor who identifies diseases by studying cells and tissues under a microscope.

pelvic: Referring to the area of the body located below the waist and surrounded by the hip and pubic bones.

pelvis: The bowl-shaped bone that supports the spine and holds up the digestive, urinary, and reproductive organs. The legs connect to the body at the pelvis.

penis (PEE-nis): The male organ used for urination and sex.

percutaneous nephrolithotomy ((PER-kyoo-TAY-nee-us NEF-roh-lih-THAH-tuh-mee): A method for removing kidney stones through keyhole surgery.

perineal prostatectomy (pe-ri-NEE-al): Surgery to remove the prostate through an incision made between the scrotum and the anus.

peripheral stem cell transplantation (per-IF-er-al): A method of replacing blood-forming cells destroyed by cancer treatment. Immature blood cells (stem cells) in the circulating blood that are similar to those in the bone marrow are given after treatment to help the bone marrow recover and continue producing healthy blood cells. Transplantation may be autologous (an individual's own blood cells saved earlier), allogeneic (blood cells donated by someone else), or syngeneic (blood cells donated by an identical twin). Also called peripheral stem cell support.

pessary (PESS-uh-ree): A specially designed object worn in the vagina to hold the bladder in its correct position and prevent leakage of urine. Pessaries come in many shapes and sizes.

Peyronie's disease (pay-ROH-neez): A plaque (hardened area) that forms on the penis, preventing that area from stretching. During erection, the penis bends in the direction of the plaque, or the plaque may lead to indentation and shortening of the penis.

prognosis (prog-NO-sis): The likely outcome or course of a disease; the chance of recovery or recurrence.

prostate (PRAH-state): In men, a walnut-shaped gland that surrounds the urethra at the neck of the bladder. The prostate supplies fluid that goes into semen.

prostate-specific antigen (PSA) (AN-tih-jen): A protein made only by the prostate gland. High levels of PSA in the blood may be a sign of prostate cancer.

prostatectomy: Surgery to remove part of the prostate. Removal of the entire prostate is called radical prostatectomy, which is performed in two ways: *Retropubic prostatectomy* is the surgical removal of the prostate through an incision in the abdomen. *Perineal prostatectomy* is surgery to remove the prostate through an incision made between the scrotum and the anus.

prostatic acid phosphatase (FOS-fa-tase): An enzyme produced by the prostate. Its level in the blood goes up in some men who have prostate cancer. Also called PAP.

prostatitis (PRAH-stuh-TY-tis): Inflammation of the prostate gland. Chronic prostatitis means the prostate gets inflamed over and over again. The most common form of prostatitis is not associated with any known infecting organism.

proteinuria (PRO-tee-NOOR-ee-uh): The presence of protein in the urine, indicating that the kidneys may not be working properly.

pyelonephritis (PY-loh-nef-RY-tis): An infection of the kidney(s), usually caused by a germ that has traveled up through the urethra, bladder, and ureter(s) from outside the body.

R

radiation oncologist (ray-dee-AY-shun on-KOL-o-jist): A doctor who specializes in using radiation to treat cancer.

radiation therapy (ray-dee-AY-shun): The use of high-energy radiation from x-rays, neutrons, and other sources to kill cancer cells and shrink tumors. Radiation may come from a machine outside the body (external-beam radiation therapy) or from material called radioisotopes. Radioisotopes produce radiation and can be placed in or near a tumor or near cancer cells. This type of radiation treatment is called internal radiation therapy, implant radiation, or brachytherapy. Systemic radiation therapy uses a radioactive substance such as a radiolabeled monoclonal antibody that circulates throughout the body. Also called radiotherapy.

radical prostatectomy: Surgery to remove the entire prostate.

radioactive (RAY-dee-o-AK-tiv): Giving off radiation.

radionuclide scanning: A test that produces pictures (scans) of internal parts of the body. The person is given an injection or swallows a small amount of radioactive material; a machine called a scanner then measures the radioactivity in certain organs.

rectal exam: A procedure in which a doctor inserts a gloved, lubricated finger into the rectum and feels the prostate through the wall of the rectum to check the prostate for hard or lumpy areas.

rectum: The last 6 to 8 inches of the large intestine. The rectum stores solid waste until it leaves the body through the anus.

recur: To occur again. Recurrence is the return of cancer, at the same site as the original (primary) tumor or in another location, after the tumor had disappeared.

remission (ree-MISH-un): Disappearance of the signs and symptoms of cancer. When this happens, the disease is said to be "in remission." Remission can be temporary or permanent.

retropubic prostatectomy (re-tro-PYOO-bik): Surgical removal of the prostate through an incision in the abdomen.

risk factor: A habit, trait, condition, or genetic alteration that increases a person's chance of developing a disease.

S

screening: Checking for disease when there are no symptoms.

scrotum (SKRO-tum): The external pouch of skin that contains the testicles.

semen: The fluid that is released through the penis during orgasm. Semen is made up of sperm from the testicles and fluid from the prostate and other sex glands.

side effects: Problems that occur when treatment affects healthy cells. Common side effects of cancer treatment are fatigue, nausea, vomiting, decreased blood cell counts, hair loss, and mouth sores.

sigmoidoscope (sig-MOY-da-skope): A thin, lighted tube used to view the inside of the colon.

sonogram (SON-o-gram): A computer picture of areas inside the body created by bouncing sound waves off organs and other tissues. Also called ultrasonogram or ultrasound.

sperm banking: Freezing sperm for use in the future. This procedure can allow men to father children after loss of fertility.

sphincter (SFINK-tur): A round muscle that opens and closes to let fluid or other matter pass into or out of an organ. Sphincter muscles keep the bladder closed until it is time to urinate.

stage: The extent of a cancer, especially whether the disease has spread from the original site to other parts of the body.

staging: Performing exams and tests to learn the extent of the cancer within the body, especially whether the disease has spread from the original site to other parts of the body.

stem cells: The cells that all blood cells come from.

stress urinary incontinence (YOOR-ih-NEHR-ee in-KON-tih-nents): Leakage of urine caused by actions—such as coughing, laughing, sneezing, running, or lifting—that place pressure on the bladder from inside the body. Stress urinary incontinence can result from either a fallen bladder or weak sphincter muscles.

surgery: A procedure to remove or repair a part of the body or to find out whether disease is present.

systemic therapy (sis-TEM-ik):Treatment that uses substances that travel through the bloodstream, reaching and affecting cells all over the body.

T

testicles (TES-ti-kuls): The two egg-shaped glands that produce sperm and male hormones.

testosterone (tes-TOS-ter-own): A male sex hormone.

tissue (TISH-oo): A group or layer of cells that are alike in type and work together to perform a specific function.

transurethral (TRANZ-yoo-REE-thrul): Through the urethra.

transurethral resection of the prostate: The use of an instrument inserted through the penis to remove tissue from the prostate. Also called TURP or TUR. Several transurethral procedures are treatments for BPH:

- *TUIP* (transurethral incision of the prostate): widens the urethra by making a few small cuts in the bladder neck, where the urethra joins the bladder, and in the prostate gland itself.

- *TUMT* (transurethral microwave thermotherapy): destroys excess prostate tissue interfering with the exit of urine from the body by using a probe in the urethra to deliver microwaves.

- *TUNA* (transurethral needle ablation): destroys excess prostate tissue with electromagnetically generated heat by using a needle-like device in the urethra.

- *TURP* (transurethral resection of the prostate): removes the excess prostate tissue by using an instrument with an electrical loop.

tumor (TOO-mer): An abnormal mass of tissue that results from excessive cell division. Tumors perform no useful body function. They may be benign (not cancerous) or malignant (cancerous).

U

ultrasound: A technique that bounces painless sound waves off organs to create an image of their structure.

urea (yoo-REE-uh): A waste product found in the blood and caused by the breakdown of protein in the liver. Urea is normally removed from the blood by the kidneys and then excreted in the urine.

ureteroscope (yoo-REE-tur-uh-scope): A tool for examining the bladder and ureters and for removing kidney stones through the urethra.

ureters (YOOR-uh-turs): Tubes that carry urine from the kidneys to the bladder.

urethra (yoo-REETH-ra): The tube that carries urine or semen to the outside of the body.

urethral obstruction: A blockage in the urethra. A kidney stone is the most common cause.

urethritis (yoo-ree-THRY-tis): Inflammation of the urethra.

urge urinary incontinence: Urinary leakage when the bladder contracts unexpectedly by itself.

uric acid stone (YOOR-ik): A kidney stone that may result from animal protein in the diet.

urinalysis (yoor-in-AL-ih-sis): A test of a urine sample that can reveal many problems of the urinary system and other body systems. The sample may be observed for physical characteristics, chemistry, the presence of drugs or germs, or other signs of disease.

urinary frequency (YOOR-ih-NEHR-ee): Urination eight or more times a day.

urinary tract: The system that takes wastes from the blood and carries them out of the body in the form of urine. The urinary tract includes the kidneys, ureters, bladder, and urethra.

urinary tract infection (UTI): An illness caused by harmful bacteria growing in the urinary tract.

urinary urgency: Inability to delay urination.

urinate (YOOR-ih-nate): To release urine from the bladder.

urine (YOOR-in): Liquid waste product filtered from the blood by the kidneys, stored in the bladder, and expelled from the body through the urethra by the act of voiding or urinating.

urodynamic tests (YOOR-oh-dy-NAM-ik):Measures of the bladder's ability to hold and release urine.

uroflow test: Measurement of the rate at which urine flows out of the body. A lower than normal rate can indicate obstruction.

urolithiasis (YOOR-oh-lih-THY-uh-sis): Stones in the urinary system.

urologist (yoo-ROL-o-jist): A doctor who specializes in diseases of the urinary organs in female and the urinary and sex organs in males.

urostomy (yoor-OSS-toh-mee): An opening through the skin to the urinary tract to allow urine to drain when normal voiding is not possible.

V

vasectomy (vas-EK-to-mee): Surgery performed to sterilize a man by cutting the vas deferens, a tube that transports sperm.

vesicoureteral reflux (VESS-ih-koh-yoo-REE-ter-ul): An abnormal condition in which urine backs up into the ureters and occasionally into the kidneys, raising the risk of infection.

void: To urinate, empty the bladder.

voiding cystourethrogram (VCUG) (SIS-toh-yoo-REE-throh-gram): An x-ray image of the bladder and urethra made during voiding. The bladder and urethra are filled with a special fluid to make the urethra clearly visible.

W

white blood cell: A type of cell in the immune system that helps the body fight infection and disease. White blood cells include lymphocytes, granulocytes, macrophages, and others.

X

x-ray: High-energy radiation used in low doses to diagnose diseases and in high doses to treat cancer.

Chapter 32

Prostate and Urologic Diseases Organizations

This chapter lists voluntary, governmental, and private organizations. Some of the organizations offer educational materials and other services to patients and the public; others primarily serve health care professionals.

Alport Syndrome Study
410 Chipeta Way
Room 156
University of Utah
Research Park
Salt Lake City, UT 84108-1297
Tel: 801-581-5479
Fax: 801-585-3232
Internet: http://www.cc.utah.edu/~cla6202/ASHP.htm

Mission: To pursue basic laboratory and clinical research, addressing the genetic basis of various forms of hereditary nephritis (Alport syndrome) with the ongoing collection of clinical family histories and laboratory samples, which are maintained in a confidential database.

Excerpted from "Directory of Kidney and Urologic Diseases Organizations," National Institute of Diabetes and Digestive and Kidney Diseases (NIDDK), 1999. Contact information updated and verified April 2001.

American Association of Clinical Urologists

1111 North Plaza Drive, Suite 550
Schaumburg, IL 60173
Tel: (847) 517-1050
Fax: (847) 517-7229

Mission: To stimulate interest in the science and practice of urology and to promote understanding of socioeconomic and political affairs affecting medical practice among clinical urologists who are members of the American Urological Association and the American Medical Association.

Materials: AACU News (bimonthly) and AACU FAX (monthly legislative update distributed by facsimile).

American Association of Genitourinary Surgeons

Department of Urology
Bowman Gray School of Medicine
Winston-Salem, NC 27157-1094
Tel: (336) 716-4131

Mission: Professional society of urologists elected into membership because of their outstanding contributions to urology.

American Association of Kidney Patients

100 South Ashley Drive, Suite 280
Tampa, FL 33602
Tel: (800) 749-2257 or (813) 223-7099
Fax: (813) 223-0001
E-Mail: AAKPnat@aol.com
Website: http://www.aakp.org
E-Mail: info@akp.org

Mission: To serve the needs and interests of kidney patients and their families. Founded by kidney patients to help others with kidney failure cope with its physical and emotional impact on their lives.

Materials: Renalife (quarterly journal) and *The Renal Flash* (monthly electronic newsletter).

American Board of Urology

2216 Ivy Road, Suite 210
Charlottesville, VA 22903
Tel: (804) 979-0059
Fax: (804) 979-0266

Mission: To identify for the public's knowledge those physicians who have satisfied the board's criteria for certification and recertification in the specialty of urology.

American Foundation for Urologic Disease
1128 North Charles Street
Baltimore, MD 21201
Toll Free: (800) 242-2383
Tel: 410-468-1800
Fax: 410-468-1808
E-Mail: admin@afud.org
Website: http://www.afud.org

Mission: To provide research grants, patient and public education and awareness, Government relations, and patient support group activities.

Materials: Informational brochure about AFUD, *Family Urology* (quarterly magazine), and patient education brochures.

American Kidney Fund
6110 Executive Boulevard, Suite 1010
Rockville, MD 20852
Tel: (800) 638-8299 or (301) 881-3052
Fax: (301) 881-0898
E-Mail: helpline@akfinc.org
Website: http://www.akfinc.org

Mission: To provide direct financial assistance, comprehensive educational programs, research grants, and community service projects for the benefit of kidney patients.

Materials: AKF Advocate, Clinical Strategies: The AKF Newsletter for Nephrology Professionals, and patient and public education brochures.

American Lithotripsy Society
305 Second Avenue, Suite 200
Waltham, MA 02451
Tel: (781) 895-9098
Fax: (781) 895-9088
E-Mail: als@lithotripsy.org
Website: http://www.lithotripsy.org

Mission: Professional membership society dedicated to addressing all aspects of lithotripsy as a medical treatment for stone disease.

Materials: ALS Quarterly News.

American Nephrology Nurses' Association
East Holly Avenue
Box 56
Pitman, NJ 08071-0056
Toll Free: 888-600-2662
Tel: 856-256-2320
Fax: 856-589-7463
Website: http://anna.inurse.com
E-Mail: anna@ajj.com

Mission: To advance the professional development of registered nurses practicing in nephrology, transplantation, and related therapies and to promote the highest standards of patient care.

Materials: ANNA Journal, ANNA Update (bimonthly newsletter), Core Curriculum for Nephrology Nursing, position statements, and clinical monographs.

American Prostate Society
7188 Ridge Road
Hanover, MD 21076
Tel: (410) 859-3735
Information line: (800) 308-1106
Fax: (410) 850-0818
Website: http://www.ameripros.org

Mission: To increase knowledge of prostate diseases and encourage the establishment of centers for diagnosis and treatment.

Materials: What You Don't Know About Your Prostate Can Kill You (brochure), Medication Versus Surgery (brochure), and quarterly newsletter.

American Society for Artificial Internal Organs Inc.
National Office
P.O. Box C
Boca Raton, FL 33429-0468
Tel: 561-391-8589
Fax: 561-368-9153
E-Mail: info@asaio.com
Website: http://www.asaio.com

Mission: ASAIO promotes the development, application, and awareness of organ technologies that enhance quality and duration of life.

Materials: ASAIO Journal (bimonthly peer-reviewed journal), *ASAIO Abstracts* (for annual conference), *ASAIO Newsletter* (quarterly newsletter on public policy education project).

American Society for Histocompatibility and Immunogenetics

P.O. Box 15804
Lenexa, KS 66285-5804
Tel: 913-541-0009
Fax: 913-541-0156
Website: http://www.ashi-hla.org

Mission: To provide investigators in the field with a mechanism for education and communication and to influence regulatory efforts, provide a forum for the exchange of research and clinical data, and offer technical workshops at an annual education meeting.

Materials: Laboratory Procedures Manual, Human Immunology Journal, membership directory, *ASHI Quarterly*.

American Society of Nephrology

2025 M Street, NW, #800
Washington, DC 20036
Tel: (202) 367-1190
Fax: (202) 367-2190
E-Mail: asn@dc.sba.com
Website: http://www.asn-online.com

Mission: To advance the knowledge and practice of nephrology.

Materials: Journal of the American Society of Nephrology (JASN) and *Highlights* (member newsletter).

American Society of Pediatric Nephrology

Rainbow Babies and Children's Hospital
11100 Euclid Avenue
Mail code 6003
Cleveland, OH 44106-6003
Tel: (216) 844-1000
Fax: (216) 844-1479
Website: http://www.uhrainbow.com

Mission: To promote public and professional educational programs in pediatric nephrology.

American Society of Transplant Surgeons
1020 North Fairfax Street, Suite 200
Alexandria, VA 22312
Tel: 888-990-2787
Fax: (202) 833-3843
E-Mail: KCrist@slackinc.com
Website: http://www.asts.org

Mission: To promote and encourage education and research with respect to organ and tissue transplantation so as to facilitate progress in the saving of lives and/or enhancing the quality of lives of patients afflicted with end stage organ failure. To collaborate with existing public and private organizations to promote and encourage education and research in transplantation and to participate and assist in the coordination of efforts or formulation of programs by all surgeons, physicians, scientists, agencies, and health personnel, which will provide maximal efficiency and optimal benefit to recipients of transplants.

American Society of Transplantation
17000 Commerce Parkway, Suite C
Mt. Laurel, NJ 08054
Tel: 856-439-9986
Fax: 856-439-9982
Website: http://www.a-s-t.org
E-Mail: ast@ahint.com

Mission: To promote and encourage education and research with respect to transplantation medicine and immunology. To provide a forum for the exchange of scientific information related to transplantation medicine and immunology. To give physicians and allied scientists interested in transplantation medicine and immunology an effective, unified, and authoritative voice in dealing with other Government, medical, and private agencies and organizations.

Materials: ASTP Newsletter (member newsletter), *ASTP Primer on Transplantation, AST Washington Roundup.*

American Urological Association Inc.
1120 North Charles Street
Baltimore, MD 21201-5559
Tel: (410) 727-1100
Fax: (410) 223-4370
E-Mail: aua@auanet.org
Website: http://www.auanet.org

Mission: To promote the highest standards of urological clinical care through education, research, and the formulation of health care policy.

Materials: Clinical practice guidelines on urological diseases.

Continence Restored Inc.
407 Strawberry Hill Avenue
Stamford, CT 06902
Tel: (914) 493-1470 (daytime) or (203) 348-0601 (evening)

Mission: To disseminate information about bladder control problems to all interested parties, to establish a network of continence support groups throughout the United States, to provide a resource for the public and professionals, and to work with manufacturers who produce incontinence products.

Council of American Kidney Societies
1444 I Street NW., Suite 700
Washington, DC 20005
Tel: (202) 712-9037
Fax: (202) 216-9646
E-Mail: caks@bostromdc.com

Mission: To serve as a representative body of scientific and professional nephrology practice organizations engaged in the promotion and support of clinical and basic research and medical practice in the broad fields of adult and pediatric kidney diseases.

Cystinuria Support Network
21001 NE 36th Street
Redmond, WA 98053
Tel: (425) 868-2996
E-Mail: Cystinuria@aol.com

Mission: To provide a resource for putting individuals in touch with each other for support and practical advice dealing with issues concerning cystinuria.

Materials: Cystinuria Support Network Newsletter.

Diabetes Insipidus and Related Disorders Network
535 Echo Court
Saline, MI 48176-1270
Tel/Fax: (734) 944-0078

Mission: To maintain a support network for patients and their families dealing with diabetes insipidus of any form; to provide emotional and informational support to those families; to educate and promote education related to diabetes insipidus; and to promote scientific research in diabetes insipidus, seeking to develop better means of treatment and ultimately scientific prevention and/or a cure.

The Diabetes Insipidus Foundation, Inc.
4533 Ridge Drive
Baltimore, MD 21229
Tel: (410) 247-3953
Fax: (410) 247-5584
E-Mail: diabetesinsipidus@maxinter.net
Website: http://diabetesinsipidus.maxinter.net

Mission: To foster improved treatment and ultimately the prevention and cure of all forms of diabetes insipidus through research, to promote a greater public awareness and understanding of the disease, and to serve patients and their families with informational material.

Materials: Endless Water (quarterly newsletter).

Hereditary Nephritis Foundation
1390 West 6690 South, #202H
Murray, UT 84123-6914
Tel/Fax: (801) 262-5901
Website: http://www.cc.utah.edu/~cla6202/HNF.htm

Mission: To promote research into the causes of and cures for hereditary nephritis and to provide up-to-date general information about Alport syndrome and related conditions to patients, families, and physicians.

Materials: HNF Newsletter (semiannual).

IgA Nephropathy Support Network
484 East State Street
Granby, MA 01033
Tel: (413) 467-9689

Mission: To assist patients with IgA nephropathy and their families; to serve as a clearinghouse for dissemination of information about IgA nephropathy; and to promote research for a possible cure.

Materials: Newsletter and pamphlets.

Impotence World Association
119 S. Ruth St
Maryville, TN 37803
Tel: (800) 669-1603
Fax: (301) 262-6825
Website: http://www.impotenceworld.org
E-Mail: info@impotenceworld.org

Mission: To inform and educate the public about impotence and its causes and treatments and to maintain a referral list of urologists who will treat and diagnose impotence.

Materials: It's Not All in Your Head (book), *Impotence Worldwide* (newsletter), various factsheets, detailed reports, and brochures.

International Pediatric Nephrology Association
c/o Montefiore Medical Center
111 E. 210th Street
Bronx, NY 10467
Tel: (718) 665-1120
Fax: (718) 652-3136

Mission: To promote professional education and improve health care for children with kidney and urologic diseases.

Materials: Pediatric Nephrology.

International Society for Peritoneal Dialysis
Georgetown University School of Medicine, F-6003-PHC
3800 Reservoir Road NW
Washington, DC 20007
Tel: (202) 784-3662
Fax: (202) 687-7893
Website: http://www.ispd.org

Mission: To advance knowledge of peritoneal dialysis.

Materials: Peritoneal Dialysis International.

International Society of Nephrology
Emory University, Renal Division
1639 Pierce Drive, WMB 338
Atlanta, GA 30322
Tel: (404) 727-8527
Fax: (404) 727-3425
Website: http://www.isn-online.org

Mission: To educate nephrologists about research and patient care.

Materials: Kidney International.

International Transplant Nurses Society
1739 E. Carson Street
Box 351
Pittsburgh, PA 15203-1700
Tel: (412) 488-0240
Fax: (412) 431-5911
Website: http://www.itns.org
E-Mail: itns@msn.com

Mission: Professional membership organization of transplant nurses dedicated to improving patient care through dissemination of information and symposia.

Materials: ITNS Newsletter.

Interstitial Cystitis Association of America, Inc. (ICA)
51 Monroe Street, Suite 1402
Rockville, MD 20850-2421
Tel: (800) HELP-ICA or (301) 610-5300
Fax: (301) 610-5308
Website: http://www.ichelp.org
E-Mail: icamail@ichelp.org

Mission: To assist patients with interstitial cystitis (IC), to educate the medical community about IC, and to promote IC research.

Materials: ICA (brochure), *ICA Update* (quarterly newsletter), transcripts of annual meetings, and patient and professional education materials.

Kidney Cancer Association
1234 Sherman Avenue
Suite 203, Evanston, IL 60202-1378
Tel: (800) 850-9132 or (847) 332-1051
Fax: (847) 332-2978
E-Mail: office@nkca.org
Website: http://www.nkca.org

Mission: To provide information to patients and physicians; to sponsor research on kidney cancer; and to act as an advocate on behalf of patients with the Federal Government, insurance companies, and employers.

Materials: We Have Kidney Cancer (56-page booklet for patients), *Kidney Cancer News* (quarterly newsletter), and public policy papers.

National Association for Continence (NAFC)
P.O. Box 8310
Spartanburg, SC 29305-8310
Tel: (800) BLADDER or (864) 579-7900
Fax: (864) 579-7902
Website: http://www.nafc.org
E-Mail: memberservices@nafc.org

Mission: To improve the quality of life for people with incontinence. NAFC is a leading source of education, advocacy, and support to the public and to the health profession about the causes, prevention, diagnosis, treatment, and management alternatives for incontinence.

Materials: Quality Care (quarterly newsletter), *The Resource Guide* (annual directory of products and services for incontinence), and assorted educational leaflets on topics related to incontinence.

National Association of Nephrology Technicians/Technologists
PO Box 2307
Dayton, OH 45401-2307
Toll Free: 877-607-6268
Tel: (937) 586-3705
Fax: (937) 586-3699
Website: http://www.dialysistech.org
E-Mail: nant@nant.meinet.com

Mission: Promote the highest quality of care for end-stage renal disease (ESRD) patients through education and professionalism by providing educational opportunities for the technical practitioner and other members of the integrated care team, representing the technical professional in the regulatory and legislative arena, developing technical professionals in leadership roles, achieving recognition for the role and significant contribution of the technical practitioner to the total care of the ESRD patient, and serving as a resource for the ESRD community to accomplish each of these goals.

Materials: Bimonthly newsletter, educational and technical manuals, regional educational meetings.

National Bladder Foundation
P.O. Box 1095
Ridgefield, CT 06877
Tel: 203-431-0005
Fax: (203) 431-0008
Website: http://www.bladder.org

Mission: To achieve the rapid discovery of cures and preventive interventions for the most common bladder diseases, through the support of research.

Materials: Patient education brochures and support-lines services.

National Foundation for Transplants (formerly the Organ Transplant Fund)
1102 Brookfield Road
Suite 200
Memphis, TN 38119
Tel: (800) 489-3863 or (901) 684-1697
Fax: (901) 684-1128
E-Mail: natfoundtx@aol.com
Website: http://www.transplants.org

Mission: To provide financial and support assistance to transplant patients and their families.

National Kidney Foundation (NKF)
30 East 33rd Street
New York, NY 10016
Tel: (800) 622-9010 or (212) 889-2210
Fax: 212-689-9261
Website: http://www.kidney.org

Mission: To prevent kidney and urinary tract diseases, improve the health and well-being of individuals and families affected by these diseases, and increase the availability of all organs for transplantation.

Materials: Advances in Renal Replacement Therapy, American Journal of Kidney Diseases, CNSW Newsletter, CRN News and Briefs (newsletter), *CNNT Newsletter, Family Focus* (newsletter), *Transplant Chronicles* (newsletter), *Journal of Renal Nutrition, Journal of Nephrology Social Work, For Those Who Give and Grieve* (newsletter), and patient and public education materials.

National Organization for Rare Disorders Inc. (NORD)
P.O. Box 8923
New Fairfield, CT 06812-8923
Tel: (203) 746-6518
Fax: (203) 746-6481
E-Mail: orphan@nord-rdb.com
Website: http://www.rarediseases.org

Mission: To act as a clearinghouse for information about rare disorders and provide a network for mutual support to match families with similar disorders; to foster communication among rare disease voluntary agencies, Government bodies, industry, scientific researchers, academic institutions, and concerned individuals; and to encourage and promote research and education about rare disorders and orphan drugs.

Materials: Fact sheets and reprints on rare disorders and *Orphan Drug Update* (newsletter).

Nephrogenic Diabetes Insipidus Foundation
Main Street
P.O. Box 1390
Eastsound, WA 98245
Tel: (888) 376-6343
Fax: (888) 376-3842
E-Mail: info@ndif.org
Website: http://www.ndif.org

Mission: To support education, research, treatment, and cure for nephrogenic diabetes insipidus. To create a communication channel to serve the entire NDI community: patients and their families, researchers, physicians, and other health care providers.

North American Transplant Coordinators Organization
P.O. Box 15384
Lenexa, KS 66285-5384
Tel: (913) 492-3600
Fax: (913) 541-0156
Website: http://www.natco1.org
E-Mail: natco-info@goAMP.com

Mission: To support, develop, and advance the knowledge of its members and enhance the quality, effectiveness, and integrity of donation and transplantation.

Materials: In Touch: Journal of Transplant Coordination and patient care brochures.

Oxalosis and Hyperoxaluria Foundation (OHF)
12 Pleasant Street
Maynard, MA 01754
Toll Free: 888-721-2432, PIN# 5392
Tel/Fax: 978-461-0614
E-Mail: info@ohf.org
Website: http://www.ohf.org

Mission: To inform the public, especially patients, parents, families, physicians, and medical professionals, about hyperoxaluria and the related conditions, i.e., oxalosis and calcium-oxalate kidney stones; to provide a support network for those affected by hyperoxaluria; and to support and encourage research to find a cure for hyperoxaluria.

Polycystic Kidney Research Foundation
4901 Main Street
Suite 200
Kansas City, MO 64112-2634
Tel: (800) PKD-CURE or (816) 931-2600
Fax: (816) 931-8655
E-Mail: pkdcure@pkdcure.org
Website: http://www.pkdcure.org

Mission: To promote research in the cause, treatment, and cure of polycystic kidney disease.

Materials: Polycystic Kidney Disease (patient manual); *PKR Progress* (quarterly newsletter); *Autosomal Recessive PKD, Questions and Answers; The Family and ADPKD;andHealth Tips for Living with PKD.*

The Prostatitis Foundation
1063 30th Street, Box 8
Smithshire, IL 61478
Tel: (888) 891-4200
Fax: (309) 325-7184
Website: http://www.prostate.org

Mission: To provide support to men with prostatitis and to push for prostatitis research funding.

Materials: The Prostatitis Foundation Information Packet.

Renal Physicians Association
4701 Randolph Road
Suite 102
Rockville, MD 20852
Tel: 301-468-3515
Fax: 301-468-3511
Website: http://www.renalmd.org
E-Mail: rpa@renalmd.org

Mission: To ensure optimal care under the highest standards of medical practice for patients with renal disease and related disorders, to act as a national representative for physicians engaged in the study and management of patients with renal disease and related disorders, and to serve as a major resource for the development of national health policy concerning renal disease.

Materials: RPA News, bimonthly, available at no cost to members; clinical practice guideline on adequacy of hemodialysis; *ESRD in the Age of Managed Care: A Primer on Capitation.*

The Simon Foundation for Continence
P.O. Box 835
Wilmette, IL 60091
Tel: (847) 864-3913
Fax: (847) 864-9758
E-Mail: simoninfo@simonfoundation.org

Website: http://www.simonfoundation.org/html/index.html

Mission: To remove the stigma from incontinence and provide help to sufferers, their families, and the professional caregiver.

Materials: The Informer (quarterly newsletter), *Managing Incontinence: A Guide to Living with the Loss of Bladder Control,* several videos, slide presentations, and other educational materials.

Society of Government Service Urologists
7027 Weathered Post
San Antonio, TX 78238
Tel: (210) 681-0587
Preston Littrell, Administrator

Mission: Professional membership organization of Government service urologists.

Society of University Urologists
PO Box 681965
San Antonio, TX 78268-7202
Website: http://www.txdirect.net/~sgsu/
E-Mail: sgsu@txdirect.net

Mission: To promote high standards in the urology field by acting as a forum for the interchange of ideas and materials relative to university urology educational programs and by fostering a balance of all phases of academic work in urology. Members consist of urologists holding faculty or teaching positions in residency training programs.

Materials: Objectives for Urology Residency Education (guidelines for educational units).

Society of Urologic Nurses and Associates
East Holly Avenue
Box 56
Pitman, NJ 08071-0056
Tel: 865-256-2332
Fax: 856-589-7463
E-Mail: suna@inurse.com
Website: http://suna.inurse.com

Mission: Professional organization committed to excellence in patient care standards and a continuum of quality care, clinical practice, and research through education of its members, patients, family, and community.

Materials: Program Newsletter, *Urologic Nursing* (official journal), and *Standards of Urologic Nursing Practice.*

The Transplant Foundation
205 Viger Avenue West
Suite 201
Montreal, QC, Canada H2Z 1G2
Tel: 514-874-1998
Fax: 514-874-1580
Website: http://www.transplantation-soc.org
E-Mail: info@transplantation-soc.org

Mission: To provide information and direct grants nationally to post-transplant recipients to offset the costs of immunosuppressive medications.

Transplant Recipients International Organization (TRIO)
1000 16th Street, NW, Suite 602
Washington, DC 20036-5705
Tel: (800) TRIO-386 or (202) 293-0980
Fax: 202-293-0973
Website: http://www.trioweb.org
E-Mail: trio@mindspring.com

Mission: TRIO is an independent, not-for-profit, international organization committed to improving the quality of life of transplant candidates, recipients, donors, and their families. Through the TRIO Headquarters and a network of chapters, TRIO serves its members in the following areas:

Awareness: Promoting organ and tissue donation as an important social responsibility. Developing and supporting mechanisms to improve availability of organs and tissues on an equitable basis to meet the needs of transplant candidates.

Support: Providing support to transplant candidates, recipients, donors, and their families to help alleviate the stresses and problems associated with the transplantation process.

Education: Providing transplant candidates, recipients, donors, and their families with current information on developments in organ and tissue donation, transplantation, medications, social issues, and finances, as well as information on initiatives in the field of transplantation by Federal, State, and local government bodies.

Advocacy: Making known to Federal, State, and local government bodies the concerns and needs that affect the welfare of transplant candidates, recipients, donors, and their families. Effectively communicating their views to the general public on issues in the field of transplantation and organ and tissue donation.

Materials: Lifelines (bimonthly), *Membership Update* (once a month for members).

United Network for Organ Sharing (UNOS)
1100 Boulders Parkway
Suite 500
P.O. Box 13770
Richmond, VA 23225
Tel: 888-TX-INFO-1 or 888-894-6361
Website: http://www.unos.org

Mission: To administer the national organ procurement and transplantation network and the national organ transplantation scientific registry under contracts with the Health Resources and Services Administration, a division of the U.S. Department of Health and Human Services. UNOS's purpose is to promote, facilitate, and scientifically advance organ procurement and transplantation and to administer an equitable organ allocation for the entire Nation. The UNOS Scientific Registry is a comprehensive organ transplantation data system enabling scientists and other interested individuals to access information for all liver, heart, heart-lung, pancreas, kidney, and small bowel donors and recipients in the United States since October 1, 1987.

Materials: UNOS Update and educational materials.

United Ostomy Association Inc. (UOA)
19772 MacArthur Boulevard ,Suite 200
Irvine, CA 92612
Tel: (800) 826-0826 or (949) 660-8624
Fax: (949) 660-9262
E-Mail: info@uoa.org
Website: http://www.uoa.org

Mission: To offer practical assistance and emotional support to ostomy patients through trained UOA members and to produce and distribute materials about ostomy care and management.

Materials: Ostomy Quarterly (magazine) and patient education materials.

National Kidney and Urologic Diseases Information Clearinghouse
3 Information Way
Bethesda, MD 20892-3580
Website: http://www.niddk.nih.gov

The National Kidney and Urologic Diseases Information Clearinghouse (NKUDIC) is a service of the National Institute of Diabetes and Digestive and Kidney Diseases (NIDDK). NIDDK is part of the National Institutes of Health under the U.S. Department of Health and Human Services. Established in 1987, the clearinghouse provides information about diseases of the kidneys and urologic system to people with kidney and urologic disorders and to their families, health care professionals, and the public. NKUDIC answers inquiries; develops, reviews, and distributes publications; and works closely with professional and patient organizations and Government agencies to coordinate resources about kidney and urologic diseases.

Chapter 33

National Organizations Offering Services to People with Cancer

People with cancer and their families sometimes need assistance coping with the emotional as well as the practical aspects of their disease. This chapter includes some of the national organizations that provide this type of support. It is not intended to be a comprehensive listing of all organizations that offer these services in the United States, nor does inclusion of any particular organization imply endorsement by the National Cancer Institute (NCI), the National Institutes of Health (NIH), or the Department of Health and Human Services (DHHS). The intent of this chapter is to provide information useful to individuals nationally. For that reason, it does not include the many local groups that offer valuable assistance to patients and their families in individual states or cities.

Alliance for Lung Cancer Advocacy, Support, and Education (ALCASE)
Post Office Box 849
Vancouver, WA 98666
Tel: 360-696-2436
Toll Free: 800-298-2436
E-Mail: info@alcase.org
Website: http://www.alcase.org

The ALCASE offers programs designed to help improve the quality of life of people with lung cancer and their families. Programs include

CancerNet, National Cancer Institute (NCI), 2000.

education about the disease, psychosocial support, and advocacy about issues that concern lung cancer survivors.

American Brain Tumor Association (ABTA)
2720 River Road
Des Plaines, IL 60018
Tel: 847-827-9910
Toll Free: 800-886-ABTA (Toll Free: 800-886-2282)
Fax: 847-827-9918
E-Mail: info@abta.org
Website: http://www.abta.org

The ABTA funds brain tumor research and provides information to help patients make educated decisions about their health care. The ABTA offers printed materials about the research and treatment of brain tumors, and provides listings of physicians, treatment facilities, and support groups throughout the country. A limited selection of Spanish-language publications is available.

American Cancer Society (ACS)
1599 Clifton Road, NE.
Atlanta, GA 30329-4251
Tel: 404-320-3333
Toll Free: 800-ACS-2345 (Toll Free: 800-227-2345)
Website: http://www.cancer.org

The ACS is a voluntary organization that offers a variety of services to patients and their families. The ACS also supports research, provides printed materials, and conducts educational programs. Staff can accept calls and distribute publications in Spanish. A local ACS unit may be listed in the white pages of the telephone directory under "American Cancer Society."

American Cancer Society (ACS) Supported Programs:

- *I Can Cope:* I Can Cope is a patient education program that is designed to help patients, families, and friends cope with the day-to-day issues of living with cancer.

- *International Association of Laryngectomies:* This program assists people who have lost their voice as a result of cancer. It provides information on the skills needed by laryngectomies and works toward total rehabilitation of patients.

- *Look Good. . .Feel Better:* This program was developed by the Cosmetic, Toiletry, and Fragrance Association Foundation in co-operation with ACS and the National Cosmetology Association. It focuses on techniques that can help people undergoing cancer treatment improve their appearance.

- *Ostomy Rehabilitation Program:* The Ostomy Rehabilitation Program provides mutual aid, emotional support, and educational materials to people with ostomies.

American Foundation for Urologic Disease

1128 North Charles Street
Baltimore, MD 21201
Toll Free: (800) 242-2383
Tel: 410-468-1800
Fax: 410-468-1808
E-Mail: admin@afud.org
Website: http://www.afud.org

The AFUD supports research; provides education to patients, the general public, and health professionals; and offers patient support services for those who have or may be at risk for a urologic disease or disorder. They provide information on urologic disease and dysfunctions, including prostate cancer treatment options, bladder health, and sexual function. They also offer prostate cancer support groups (Prostate Cancer Network). Some Spanish-language publications are available.

American Institute for Cancer Research (AICR)

1759 R Street, NW.
Washington, DC 20009
Tel: 202-328-7744
Toll Free: 800-843-8114
E-Mail: aicrweb@aicr.org
Website: http://www.aicr.org

The AICR provides information about cancer prevention, particularly through diet and nutrition. They offer a toll-free nutrition hotline, pen pal support network, funding of research grants, and a wide array of consumer and health professional brochures and health aids about diet and nutrition and its link to cancer and cancer prevention. The AICR also offers the AICR CancerResource, an information and resource program for cancer patients. A limited selection of Spanish-language publications is available.

275

The Brain Tumor Society
124 Watertown St., Suite 3H
Watertown, MA 02472
Tel: 617-924-9997
Toll Free: 800-770-TBTS
Fax: 617-924-9998
E-Mail: info@tbts.org
Website: http://www.tbts.org

The Brain Tumor Society provides information about brain tumors and related conditions for patients and their families. They offer a patient/family telephone network, educational publications, funding for research projects, and access to support groups for patients.

Cancer Care, Inc.
275 Seventh Avenue
New York, NY 10001
Tel: 212-302-2400
Toll Free: 800-813-HOPE (Toll Free: 800-813-4673)
E-Mail: info@cancercare.org
Website: http://www.cancercare.org

Cancer Care provides free, professional assistance to people with any type of cancer, at any stage of illness, and to their families. This organization offers education, one-on-one counseling, specialized support groups, financial assistance for nonmedical expenses, home visits by trained volunteers, and referrals to community services. A section of the Cancer Care Web site and some publications are available in Spanish, and staff can respond to calls and e-mails in Spanish.

Cancer Hope Network
Two North Road
Suite A
Chester, NJ 07930
Tel: 1-877-HOPENET (1-877-467-3638)
E-Mail: info@cancerhopenetwork.org
Website: http://www.cancerhopenetwork.org

Cancer Hope Network provides individual support to cancer patients and their families by matching them with trained volunteers who have undergone and recovered from a similar cancer experience. Such matches are based on the type and stage of cancer, treatments used, side effects experienced, and other factors.

Cancer Research Foundation of America
1600 Duke Street
Suite 110
Alexandria, VA 22314
Tel: 703-836-4412
Toll Free: 800-227-2732
Fax: 703-836-4413
Website: http://www.preventcancer.org

The Cancer Research Foundation of America seeks to prevent cancer through funding research and providing educational materials on early detection and nutrition.

Candlelighters Childhood Cancer Foundation (CCCF)
3910 Warner Street
Kensington, MD 20895
Tel: 301-962-3520
Toll Free: 800-366-CCCF (Toll Free: 800-366-2223)
E-Mail: info@candlelighters.org
Website: http://www.candlelighters.org

The CCCF is a nonprofit organization that provides information, peer support, and advocacy through publications, an information clearing-house, and a network of local support groups. A financial aid list is available listing organizations to which eligible families may apply for assistance.

CaP CURE (Association for the Cure of Cancer of the Prostate)
1250 Fourth Street
Suite 360
Santa Monica, CA 90401
Tel: 310-458-2873
Toll Free: 800-757-CURE (Toll Free: 800-757-2873)
E-Mail: capcure@capcure.org
Website: http://www.capcure.org

CaP CURE is a nonprofit organization that provides funding for re-search projects to improve methods of diagnosing and treating pros-tate cancer. It also offers printed resources for prostate cancer survivors and their families. The mission of CaP CURE is to find a cure for prostate cancer.

Children's Hospice International
2202 Mount Vernon Avenue, Suite 3C
Alexandria, VA 22301
Tel: 703-684-0330
Toll Free: 800-2-4-CHILD (Toll Free: 800-242-4453)
Fax: 703-684-0226
E-Mail: chiorg@aol.com
Website: http://www.chionline.org

Children's Hospice International provides a network of support for dying children and their families. It serves as a clearinghouse for research programs and support groups, and offers educational materials and training programs on pain management and the care of seriously ill children.

Cure For Lymphoma Foundation (CFL)
215 Lexington Avenue
New York, NY 10016-6023
Tel: 212-213-9595
Toll Free: 800-CFL-6848 (Toll Free: 800-235-6848)
Fax: 212-213-1987
E-Mail: infocfl@cfl.org
Website: http://www.cfl.org

The CFL offers support and education programs and services to patients and caregivers. Materials and services include: "Understanding Lymphoma" booklets and fact sheets; lymphoma family forums; teleconferences; lymphoma Q & A's; a nationwide Patient-to-Patient Telephone Network; bi-weekly support groups; monthly lymphoma networking groups; patient aid; quarterly newsletter, *Together*; and a toll-free information line. CFL also funds lymphoma research and collaborates with researchers, clinicians, social workers, and nurses. The CFL works to increase public awareness of lymphoma through grassroots public education campaigns.

HOSPICELINK
Hospice Education Institute
190 Westbrook Road
Essex, CT 06426-1510
Tel: 860-767-1620
Toll Free: 800-331-1620
Fax: 860-767-2746
E-Mail: HOSPICEALL@aol.com
Website: http://www.hospiceworld.org

HOSPICELINK helps patients and their families find support services in their communities. They offer information about hospice and palliative care and can refer cancer patients and their families to local hospice and palliative programs.

International Myeloma Foundation (IMF)
12650 Riverside Drive, Suite 206
North Hollywood, CA 91607
Tel: 818-487-7455
Toll Free: 800-452-CURE (Toll Free: 800-452-2873)
Fax: 818-487-7475
E-Mail: TheIMF@myeloma.org
Website: http://www.myeloma.org

IMF supports education, treatment, and research for multiple myeloma. They provide a toll-free hotline, seminars, and educational materials for patients and their families. Although the IMF does not sponsor support groups, they do keep a list of other organizations' support groups and provide information on how to start a support group. A section of the IMF Web site and some printed materials are available in Spanish.

Kidney Cancer Association
1234 Sherman Avenue, Suite 203
Evanston, IL 60202-1375
Tel: 847-332-1051
Toll Free: 800-850-9132
Fax: 847-332-2978
E-Mail: office@nkca.org
Website: http://www.nkca.org

The Kidney Cancer Association supports research, offers printed materials about the diagnosis and treatment of kidney cancer, sponsors support groups, and provides physician referral information.

The Leukemia and Lymphoma Society
1311 Mamaroneck Avenue
White Plains, NY 10605-5221
Tel: 914-949-5213
Toll Free: 800-955-4572
Fax: 914-949-6691
E-Mail: infocenter@leukemia-lymphoma.org
Website: http://www.leukemia-lymphoma.org

The goal of the Leukemia and Lymphoma Society is to find cures for leukemia, lymphoma, Hodgkin's disease and myeloma and to improve the quality of life of patients and their families. The Society supports medical research and provides health education materials, as well as the following services: patient financial aid for specified treatment expenses and transportation, family support groups, First Connection (a professionally supervised peer support program), referrals, school re-entry materials, and public and professional education. The Society also provides audiotapes in English and some Spanish-language publications.

Lymphoma Research Foundation of America (LRFA)
8800 Venice Boulevard, Suite 207
Los Angeles, CA 90034
Tel: 310-204-7040
Toll Free: 800-500-9976
Fax: 310-204-7043
E-Mail: LRFA@aol.com
Website: http://www.lymphoma.org

LRFA funds research and provides educational information on lymphoma. They offer a helpline for general information on lymphoma, as well as referrals to other resources, oncologists, clinical trials, and support groups. A buddy program is available to match newly diagnosed patients with other lymphoma patients who have coped with the disease. Some Spanish-language publications are available.

Multiple Myeloma Research Foundation (MMRF)
11 Forest Street
New Canaan, CT 06840
Tel: 203-972-1250
E-Mail: themmrf@themmrf.org
Website: http://www.multiplemyeloma.org

MMRF supports research grants ad professional and patient symposia on multiple myeloma and related blood cancers. MMRF publishes a quarterly newsletter, and provides referrals and information packets free of charge to patients and family members.

National Brain Tumor Foundation (NBTF)
414 Thirteenth Street, Suite 700
Oakland, CA 94612-2603
Tel: 510-839-9777

Toll Free: 800-934-CURE (Toll Free: 800-934-2873)
E-Mail: nbtf@braintumor.org
Website: http://www.braintumor.org

NBTF provides patients and their families with information on how to cope with their brain tumors. This organization conducts national and regional conferences; publishes printed materials for patients and family members; provides access to a national network of patient support groups; and assists in answering patient inquiries. NBTF also awards grants to fund research. Staff are available to answer calls in Spanish, and some Spanish-language publications are available.

National Childhood Cancer Foundation (NCCF)
440 East Huntington Drive
Post Office Box 60012
Arcadia, CA 91066-6012
Tel: 626-447-1674
Toll Free: 800-458-6223
Fax: 626-445-4334
E-Mail: nccf-info@nccf.org
Website: http://www.nccf.org

The NCCF supports research conducted by a network of institutions, each of which has a team of doctors, scientists, and other specialists with the special skills required for the diagnosis, treatment, supportive care, and research on the cancers of infants, children, and young adults. Advocating for children with cancer and the centers that treat them is also a focus of the NCCF. A limited selection of Spanish-language publications is available.

National Coalition for Cancer Survivorship (NCCS)
1010 Wayne Avenue
Suite 770
Silver Spring, MD 20910-5600
Tel: 301-650-9127
Toll Free: 877-NCCS-YES (1-877-622-7937)
Fax: 301-565-9670
E-Mail: info@cansearch.org
Website: http://www.cansearch.org

NCCS is a network of groups and individuals that offer support to cancer survivors and their loved ones. It provides information and resources on cancer support, advocacy, and quality of life issues. A section of the NCCS Web site and a limited selection of publications are available in Spanish.

National Hospice and Palliative Care Organization (NHPCO)
1700 Diagonal Road
Suite 300
Alexandria, VA 22314
Tel: 703-243-5900
Toll Free: 800-658-8898 (Helpline)
E-Mail: helpline@nhpco.org
Website: http://www.nhpco.org

The NHPCO is an association of programs that provide hospice and palliative care. It is designed to increase awareness about hospice services and to champion the rights and issues of terminally ill patients and their family members. They offer discussion groups, publications, information about how to find a hospice, and information about the financial aspects of hospice. Some Spanish-language publications are available, and staff are able to answer calls in Spanish.

National Lymphedema Network (NLN)
1611 Telegraph Avenue
Suite 1111
Oakland, CA 94612-2138
Tel: 510-208-3200
Toll Free: 800-541-3259
Fax: 510-208-3110
E-Mail: nln@lymphnet.org
Website: http://www.lymphnet.org

The NLN provides education and guidance to lymphedema patients, health care professionals, and the general public by disseminating information on the prevention and management of primary and secondary lymphedema. They provide a toll-free support hotline, a referral service to lymphedema treatment centers and health care professionals, a quarterly newsletter with information about medical and scientific developments, support groups, pen pals, educational courses for health care professionals and patients, and a computer database. Some Spanish-language materials are available.

National Marrow Donor Program
3001 Broadway Street, NE, Suite 500
Minneapolis, MN 55413
Tel: 612-627-5800
Toll Free: 800-MARROW-2 (Toll Free: 800-627-7692)
888-999-6743 (Office of Patient Advocacy)
Website: http://www.marrow.org

The National Marrow Donor Program, which is funded by the Federal Government, was created to improve the effectiveness of the search for bone marrow donors. It keeps a registry of potential bone marrow donors and provides free information on bone marrow transplantation, peripheral blood stem cell transplant and unrelated donor stem cell transplant including the use of umbilical cord blood.

Pancreatic Cancer Action Network (PanCAN)
Post Office Box 1010
Torrence, CA 90505
Tel: 1-877-2-PANCAN (1-877-272-6226)
Fax: 310-791-5224
E-Mail: information@pancan.org
Website: http://www.pancan.org

PanCAN, a nonprofit advocacy organization, educates health professionals and the general public about pancreatic cancer to increase awareness of the disease. PanCAN also advocates for increased funding of pancreatic cancer research and promotes access to and awareness of the latest medical advances, support networks, clinical trials, and reimbursement for care.

Patient Advocate Foundation (PAF)
753 Thimble Shoals Boulevard, Suite B
Newport News, VA 23606
Tel: 757-873-6668
Toll Free: 800-532-5274
Fax: 757-873-8999
E-Mail: help@patientadvocate.org
Website: http://www.patientadvocate.org

The PAF provides education, legal counseling, and referrals to cancer patients and survivors concerning managed care, insurance, financial issues, job discrimination, and debt crisis matters.

R. A. Bloch Cancer Foundation, Inc.
4435 Main Street
Suite 500
Kansas City, MO 64111
Tel: 816-WE-BUILD (816-932-8453)
Toll Free: 800-433-0464
Fax: 816-931-7486
E-Mail: hotline@hrblock.com
Website: http://www.blochcancer.org

The R. A. Bloch Cancer Foundation matches newly diagnosed cancer patients with trained, home-based volunteers who have been treated for the same type of cancer. They also distribute informational materials, including a multidisciplinary list of institutions that offer second opinions. Information is available in Spanish.

The Skin Cancer Foundation
245 5th Avenue, Suite 1403
New York, NY 10016
Toll Free: 800-SKIN-490 (Toll Free: 800-754-6490)
Fax: 212-725-5751
E-Mail: info@skincancer.org
Website: http://www.skincancer.org

Major goals of the Skin Cancer Foundation are to increase public awareness of the importance of taking protective measures against the damaging rays of the sun and to teach people how to recognize the early signs of skin cancer. They conduct public and medical education programs to help reduce skin cancer.

STARBRIGHT Foundation
11835 West Olympic Blvd.
Suite 500
Los Angeles, CA 90064
Tel: 310-479-1212
Fax: 310-479-1235
Website: http://www.starbright.org

The STARBRIGHT Foundation creates projects that are designed to help seriously ill children and adolescents cope with the psychosocial and medical challenges they face. The STARBRIGHT Foundation produces materials such as interactive educational CD-ROMs and videos about medical conditions and procedures, advice on talking with a health professional, and other issues related to children and adolescents who have serious medical conditions. All materials are available to children, adolescents, and their families free of charge. Staff can respond to calls in Spanish.

United Ostomy Association Inc. (UOA)
19772 MacArthur Boulevard
Suite 200
Irvine, CA 92612
Tel: (800) 826-0826 or (949) 660-8624
Fax: (949) 660-9262
E-Mail: info@uoa.org
Website: http://www.uoa.org

The United Ostomy Association helps ostomy patients through mutual aid and emotional support. It provides information to patients and the public and sends volunteers to visit with new ostomy patients.

US TOO International, Inc.
5003 Fairview Avenue
Downers Grove, IL 60515
Tel: 630-795-1002
Toll Free: 800-80-US TOO (Toll Free: 800-808-7866)
Fax: 630-795-1602
E-Mail: ustoo@ustoo.com
Website: http://www.ustoo.com

US TOO is a prostate cancer support group organization. Goals of US TOO are to increase awareness of prostate cancer in the community, educate men newly diagnosed with prostate cancer, offer support groups, and provide the latest information about treatment for this disease. A limited selection of Spanish-language publications is available.

The Wellness Community
35 East Seventh Street
Suite 412
Cincinnati, OH 45202
Tel: 513-421-7111
Toll Free: 888-793-WELL (1-888-793-9355)
Fax: 513-421-7119
E-Mail: help@wellness-community.org
Website: http://www.wellness-community.org

The Wellness Community provides free psychological and emotional support to cancer patients and their families. They offer support groups facilitated by licensed therapists, stress reduction and cancer education workshops, nutrition guidance, exercise sessions, and social events.

Vital Options and "The Group Room" Cancer Radio Talk Show
Post Office Box 19233
Encino, CA 91416-9233
Tel: 818-508-5657
Toll Free: 800-GRP-ROOM (Toll Free: 800-477-7666)
E-Mail: info@vitaloptions.org
Website: http://www.vitaloptions.org

The mission of Vital Options is to use communications technology to reach people dealing with cancer. This organization holds a weekly syndicated call-in cancer radio talk show called "The Group Room," which provides a forum for patients, long-term survivors, family members, physicians, and therapists to discuss cancer issues. Listeners can participate in the show during its broadcast every Sunday from 4 p.m.-6 p.m., ET by calling either of the telephone numbers. A live Web simulcast of "The Group Room" can be heard by logging onto the Vital Options Web site.

Chapter 34

Finding Cancer Support Groups

People with cancer and their families face many challenges that may leave them feeling overwhelmed, afraid, and alone. Sometimes it can be difficult to cope with these challenges or to talk to even the most supportive family and friends. However, members of the health care team and support groups can help the person feel less alone and can improve their ability to deal with the uncertainties and challenges cancer brings.

How can support groups help?

People with cancer sometimes find they need assistance coping with the emotional as well as the practical aspects of their disease. In fact, attention to the emotional burden of having cancer is sometimes part of a patient's treatment plan. Cancer support groups are designed to provide a confidential atmosphere where cancer patients or cancer survivors can discuss the challenges that accompany the illness with others who may be having similar experiences. For example, people gather to discuss the emotional needs created by cancer, to exchange information about their disease, including practical problems such as getting to and from treatment or managing side effects, and to share their feelings. Support groups have helped thousands of people cope with these and similar situations.

Excerpted from "Questions and Answers about Finding Cancer Support Groups," Fact Sheet 8.8, National Cancer Institute (NCI), 1997; and from "How to Find Resources in Your Own Community If You Have Cancer," Fact Sheet 8.9, National Cancer Institute, 2000.

Can family members and friends participate in support groups?

Family and friends are also affected when cancer touches someone they love. In addition to supporting the person with cancer, family members and friends may need help in dealing with stresses such as family disruptions, financial worries, and changing roles within the family. To help meet these needs, some support groups are designed just for family members of people with cancer; other groups encourage families and friends to participate with the patient.

How can people find support groups?

Many organizations offer support groups for individuals with cancer and family members or friends of those who are ill. The doctor, nurse, or hospital social worker will have information about support groups, such as their location, size, type, and how often they meet. Moreover, most hospitals have social services departments that provide information about cancer support programs. Many newspapers carry a special health supplement containing information about where to find support groups.

What types of support groups are available?

There are several kinds of support groups to meet individual needs. Support groups may be led by a professional, such as a psychiatrist, psychologist, or social worker, or by other patients. These groups may be for a particular disease (for example, for prostate cancer patients), for teens or young adults, for family members, or for more general support. Many groups are free, but some require a fee (check to see if insurance will cover the cost). In addition, support groups can vary in approach, size, and how often they meet. It is important that individuals find an atmosphere that they are comfortable with and meets their individual needs

How to Find Resources in Your Own Community If You have Cancer

If you have cancer or are undergoing cancer treatment, there are places in your community to turn to for help. There are many local organizations throughout the country that offer a variety of practical and support services to people with cancer. However, people often don't know about these services or are unable to find them. National cancer organizations can assist you in finding these resources, and there are a number of things you can do for yourself.

Whether you are looking for a support group, counseling, advice, financial assistance, transportation to and from treatment, or information about cancer, most neighborhood organizations, local health care providers, or area hospitals are a good place to start. Often, the hardest part of looking for help is knowing the right questions to ask.

What Kind of Help Can I Get?

Until now, you probably never thought about the many issues and difficulties that arise with a diagnosis of cancer. There are support services to help you deal with almost any type of problem that might occur. The first step in finding the help you need is knowing what types of services are available.

Information on Cancer

Most national cancer organizations provide a range of information services, including materials on different types of cancer, treatments, and treatment-related issues.

Counseling

While some people are reluctant to seek counseling, studies show that having someone to talk to reduces stress and helps people both mentally and physically. Counseling can also provide emotional support to cancer patients and help them better understand their illness. Different types of counseling include individual, group, family, self-help (sometimes called peer counseling), bereavement, patient-to-patient, and sexuality.

Medical Treatment Decisions

Often, people with cancer need to make complicated medical decisions. Many organizations provide hospital and physician referrals for second opinions and information on clinical trials (research studies with people), which may expand treatment options.

Prevention and Early Detection

While cancer prevention may never be 100 percent effective, many things (such as quitting smoking and eating healthy foods) can greatly reduce a person's risk for developing cancer. Prevention services usually focus on smoking cessation and nutrition. Early detection services, which are designed to detect cancer when a person has no symptoms of disease, can include referrals for screening mammograms, Pap tests, or prostate exams.

Home Health Care

Home health care assists patients who no longer need to stay in a hospital or nursing home, but still require professional medical help. Skilled nursing care, physical therapy, social work services, and nutrition counseling are all available at home.

Hospice Care

Hospice is care focused on the special needs of terminally ill cancer patients. Sometimes called palliative care, it centers around providing comfort, controlling physical symptoms, and giving emotional support to patients who can no longer benefit from curative treatment. Hospice programs provide services in various settings, including the patient's home, hospice centers, hospitals, or skilled nursing facilities. Your doctor or social worker can provide a referral for these services.

Rehabilitation

Rehabilitation services help people adjust to the effects of cancer and its treatment. Physical rehabilitation focuses on recovery from the physical effects of surgery or the side effects associated with chemotherapy. Occupational or vocational therapy helps people readjust to everyday routines, get back to work, or find employment.

Advocacy

Advocacy is a general term that refers to promoting or protecting the rights and interests of a certain group, such as cancer patients.

Advocacy groups may offer services to assist with legal, ethical, medical, employment, legislative, or insurance issues, among others. For instance, if you feel your insurance company has not handled your claim fairly, you may want to advocate for a review of its decision.

Financial

Having cancer can be a tremendous financial burden to cancer patients and their families. There are programs sponsored by the Government and nonprofit organizations to help cancer patients with problems related to medical billing, insurance coverage, and reimbursement issues. There are also sources for financial assistance, and ways to get help collecting entitlements from Medicaid, Medicare, and the Social Security Administration.

Housing/Lodging

Some organizations provide lodging for the family of a patient undergoing treatment, especially if it is a child who is ill and the parents are required to accompany the child to treatment.

Children's Services

A number of organizations provide services for children with cancer, including summer camps, make-a-wish programs, and help for parents seeking child care.

How to Find These Services

Often, the services that people with cancer are looking for are right in their own neighborhood or city. The following is a list of places where you can begin your search for help.

The hospital, clinic, or medical center where you see your doctor, received your diagnosis, or where you undergo treatment should be able to give you information. Your doctor or nurse may be able to tell you about your specific medical condition, pain management, rehabilitation services, home nursing, or hospice care.

Most hospitals also have a social work, home care, or discharge planning department. This department may be able to help you find a support group, a nonprofit agency that helps people who have cancer, or the government agencies that oversee Social Security, Medicare, and Medicaid. While you are undergoing treatment, be sure to ask the hospital about transportation, practical assistance, or even temporary child care. Talk to a hospital financial counselor in the business office about developing a monthly payment plan if you need help with hospital expenses.

The public library is an excellent source of information, as are patient libraries at many cancer centers. A librarian can help you find books and articles through a literature search.

A local church, synagogue, YMCA or YWCA, or fraternal order may provide financial assistance, or may have volunteers who can help with transportation and home care. Catholic Charities, the United Way, or the American Red Cross may also operate local offices. Some of these organizations may provide home care, and the United Way's information and referral service can refer you to an agency that provides financial help. To find the United Way serving your community, visit their online directory at http://www.unitedway.org on the Internet or look in the White Pages of your local telephone book.

Local or county government agencies may offer low-cost transportation (sometimes called para-transit) to individuals unable to use public transportation. Most states also have an Area Agency on Aging that offers low-cost services to people over 60. Your hospital or community social worker can direct you to government agencies for entitlements, including Social Security, state disability, Medicaid, income maintenance, and food stamps. (Keep in mind that most applications to entitlement programs take some time to process.) The Federal government also runs the Hill-Burton program (1–800–638–0742), which funds certain medical facilities and hospitals to provide cancer patients with free or low-cost care if they are in financial need.

Getting the Most from a Service: What to Ask

No matter what type of help you are looking for, the only way to find resources to fit your needs is to ask the right questions. When you are calling an organization for information, it is important to think about what questions you are going to ask before you call. Many people find it helpful to write out their questions in advance, and to take notes during the call. Another good tip is to ask the name of the person with whom you are speaking in case you have followup questions. Following are some of the questions you may want to consider if you are calling or visiting a new agency and want to learn about how they can help:

- How do I apply [for this service]?
- Are there eligibility requirements? What are they?
- Is there an application process? How long will it take? What information will I need to complete the application process?
- Will I need anything else to get the service?
- Do you have any other suggestions or ideas about where I can find help?

The most important thing to remember is that you will rarely receive help unless you ask for it. In fact, asking can be the hardest part of getting help. Don't be afraid or ashamed to ask for assistance. Cancer is a very difficult disease, but there are people and services that can ease your burdens and help you focus on your treatment and recovery.

Chapter 35

Managing Insurance Issues

What You Can Expect

If you are like most cancer survivors, the costs of initial treatment and continuing care are a major concern. What happens to insurance coverage and costs after you've had treatment for cancer?

In general, people who had life and health insurance before treatment are able to keep it, although costs and benefits may changes. Those who change jobs or apply for new policies, however, often face problems.

The stories of the following cancer survivors show common post-treatment insurance experiences.

"I'm grateful my insurance benefits are safe at my company. I only wish my job had more going for it. I'm working hard to find something that pays better and offers more growth. But along with finding the right job, I'm also looking for a good benefits package that is fully open to a cancer survivor. So far, the two haven't come together."

—Ron L.

"I never even thought about life insurance before I got cancer. My wife and I are young, and we had enough expenses. But after my diagnosis, I felt like I should get some insurance for my

---

Excerpted from "Managing Insurance Issues," CancerNet, National Cancer Institute (NCI), 2000.

wife's sake. It turned out to be harder than I'd expected. Several companies refused to accept me at all. I have coverage now, but the policy has an 'exclusion' for cancer, and it pays nothing if cancer is the cause of death. My doctor says it's very unlikely that my cancer will recur. But I'm still looking for another policy where having had cancer doesn't hurt me."

—Burt W.

"I knew I had health insurance, but I had no idea what it covered. And when I went into the hospital, the last thing on my mind was the cost of the treatment. When the bills started coming in, I was shocked that my company's insurance policy didn't cover everything. At first, I felt like everything about my health had gone out of my control, but I started to take charge again by learning about the claims process and pleading my own case."

—Bill G.

"My insurance company paid for all of my cancer care, but my radiation treatment made me unable to father a child. When my wife and I looked into artificial insemination, we found that insurance would not cover the cost of donor sperm. We decided to adopt a child instead."

—Brian K.

"When my health insurance company canceled my individual policy after my cancer treatment, I started checking into other options. My best bet turned out to be joining my new company's group policy, even though employees have to pay all their own premiums. The benefits are pretty good, and they accepted me despite the cancer history. But I had to fill out a health history and have a physical exam that none of my coworkers had to complete. There was also a 5-year 'waiting period' before I could submit any bills for cancer care. Luckily, I got through 5 years with no major expenses."

—Jean T.

"I had been covered under my husband's health insurance policy, and we had no problems until he changed jobs. When the new company saw my cancer history, they denied him family coverage. I was finally able to get insurance through my state health insurance pool."

—Laura S.

"My health insurance after cancer treatment worked pretty much like my car insurance: After I had an accident, my rates went up."

—*Barbara K.*

Tips for Making the Most of Your Insurance

Get all the benefits your policy provides.

- Get a copy of your insurance policies and find out exactly what your coverage includes.

- Keep careful records of all your covered expenses and claims.

- File claims for all covered costs. Surprisingly, many cancer survivors don't take full advantage of their insurance, either because they don't know about a benefit or are confused or put off by the paperwork.

- Get help in filing a claim if you need it. If friends or family can't assist, ask a social worker for help. Private companies and some community organizations also offer insurance filing aid.

- If your claim is turned down, file again. Ask your doctor to explain to the company why the services meet the requirements for coverage under your policy. If you are turned down again, find out if the company has an appeals process.

Keep insurance needs in mind when you are changing job status.

- Don't leave a job with insurance benefits until you have a new job with good coverage or you have made other plans for insurance. This is also an important thing for your spouse to keep in mind if you are covered under his or her policy.

- Look at the differences in insurance coverage and other benefits offered by various employers. You may be better off taking a new job with a lower salary that has better insurance coverage.

Consider continuing to take part in your current company's group plan after you leave. If a new job does not work out, you could be left with no coverage. Federal law (Public Law 99-272), the Consolidated Omnibus Budget Reconciliation Act (COBRA), requires many employers to allow employees who quit, are let go, or whose hours are reduced to pay their own premiums for the company's group plan. This protection lasts 18 months for employees (up to 29 months if they lose their jobs due to disability and are eligible for Social Security disability benefits at the time they leave the job) and 36 months for their dependents. If an employee leaves a company and takes a new job, continuation coverage by the former company can be kept for up to 18 months if the new company's coverage is limited or excludes a pre-existing condition, such as cancer. (COBRA applies to employers with 20 or more workers who already offer group health insurance.) Contact your personnel department to enroll. In addition, you can contact your state insurance commissioner to learn if your state has continuation-of-benefits laws. They may help you receive additional insurance rights protection.

- Take advantage of your right in some company group policies to convert to an individual policy when you leave the company or retire. Typically, a cancer survivor can obtain coverage for about a year under a converted policy. Premiums for individual policies, however, may be considerably higher and less comprehensive. You may want to check around with different companies for the best coverage at the lowest rates because each may have a different system for assessing premiums.

- Look for work in a large company, whose group insurance plans rarely exclude employees with a history of illness.

- Work with your doctors to get maximum coverage of clinical trials' costs.

Many clinical trials (treatment studies) offer some part of care free of charge. But some insurers will not cover certain costs when a new treatment is under study. If you are taking part in or considering a clinical trial:

- Ask your doctor about the experience of other patients in the trial. Have their insurers paid for their care? Have there been any consistent problems?

- Talk to your doctor about the paperwork he or she submits to your insurer. Often the way the doctor describes a treatment can help or hurt your chances of insurance coverage.

- Be sure you know what's in your policy. Check it to see if there's a specific exclusion for "experimental treatment."

Many companies handle new treatments on a case-by-case basis, rather than having a blanket policy. You always can ask about their coverage of specific therapies. However, some patients say that their questions may have hurt their chances for coverage by raising a red flag.

Find ways to supplement your insurance.

Take all the Federal income tax deductions for health care costs that you are allowed. Examples include gas mileage for trips to and from medical appointments, out-of-pocket costs for prescription drugs and equipment, and meals during lengthy medical visits.

What Your Health Insurance Coverage Should Include

When looking into a new health insurance plan, it's a good idea to make sure that the coverage provided suits your health care needs. Health insurance for the cancer survivor should provide, at the very least, the following:

- *Benefits.* Inpatient hospital care, physician services, laboratory and x ray services, prenatal care, inpatient psychiatric care, outpatient services, and nursing home care. Prescription drug coverage may be important if you will be taking a medicine for a long time.

- *Financial protection.* The insurer should pay at least 80 percent of the covered services, except for inpatient psychiatric care, which may require that the policyholder pay more than 20 percent of expenses. In addition, the insurer should pay at least $250,000 for catastrophic illness coverage, with the patient paying no more than 30 percent of his or her income toward these expenses.

Confirm conversations with insurance representatives in writing. If you think the representative is wrong, ask to speak with his/her supervisor.

Consider filing an insurance complaint if you feel you have been treated unfairly.

- If your insurer is a private company (e.g., Blue Cross, Prudential), it is regulated by your state department of Insurance.

- If your insurer is a licensed health care service plan (e.g., Kaiser and other HMOs), it is regulated by your state department of insurance.

- If your insurer is a federal qualified Health Maintenance Organization, it is regulated by the U.S. Health Care Financing Administration, Office of Prepaid Health Care Operations and Oversight.

- If your insurer is a private employer or union self-insurance or a self-financed plan, it is regulated by the U.S. Department of Labor, Pension & Welfare Benefits Administration.

- If your insurer is Medicaid (sometimes called other names; e.g., in California it's known as MediCal), it is regulated by your state department of social services or medical assistance services.

- If your insurer is Medicare, it is regulated by the U.S. Social Security Administration.

- If your insurer is Supplemental Security Income, it is regulated by the U.S. Social Security Administration.

- If your insurer is Veterans Benefits, it is regulated by the Department of Veterans Affairs, Veterans Assistance Service.

- If your insurer is CHAMPUS, it is regulated by the Department of Veterans Affairs, Veterans Assistance Service.

Options for Getting Insurance after Cancer Treatment

- Obtain dependent coverage under your spouse's insurance plan.

- Join your current company plan.

- Join a health maintenance organization. Look for open enrollment periods when you may be accepted regardless of your health history.

- Request group insurance through a professional, fraternal, membership, or political organization to which you belong.

- Use Medicare. It covers most people age 65 or older and those who are permanently disabled.

- Use Medicaid or other state or local benefits. Coverage and eligibility criteria differ from state to state; check with your local office.

- Get coverage through an independent broker.

- Join a state "high risk" health insurance pool for people who cannot get conventional coverage.

States That Provide Health Insurance Coverage for the Hard-To-Insure

A number of states currently sell comprehensive health insurance to state residents with serious medical conditions who can't find a company to insure them. Call directory assistance in your state capital for contact information.

Additional Resources

Many people need help paying for medical costs that aren't covered by their insurance. For financial assistance, you may want to contact:

Local Groups

- Local cancer support organizations, which may provide referrals to community sources for financial aid.

- Your local office on aging, if you are an older adult.

- The county board of assistance or welfare office.

United States Government

The U. S. Government has a number of programs designed to help people with low incomes or disabilities pay their bills. For information, call your local office of:

- *Aid to Families With Dependent Children (AFDC) and Food Stamps Programs.* Look for the numbers under the Local Government, Social Services, section of your telephone book.

- *Medicare/Medicaid Information.* Call your local Social Security Administration office to receive an explanation of the medical costs covered by these Federal health insurance programs. Note: For people under age 65, Medicare coverage does not begin until 2 years from the date they are declared disabled.

- *Social Security Administration.* Call 1-800-772-1213 for general information on Social Security benefits you may be eligible to receive.

- *The Department of Veterans Affairs.* Request information about medical benefits for veterans and their dependents.

- *The Cancer Information Service of the National Cancer Institute.* Call 1-800-4 CANCER to request information about drug companies with assistance programs for cancer patients with low incomes.

Your Hospital

Financial help may also be available within hospitals. To find out about setting up monthly payment plans for hospital bills, contact your:

- Hospital patient advocate.

- Hospital financial aid counselor.

- Hospital social worker.

- Patient representative in the hospital business office.

Chapter 36

Financial Assistance for Cancer Care

Cancer imposes heavy economic burdens on both patients and their families. For many people, a portion of medical expenses is paid by their health insurance plan. For individuals who do not have health insurance or who need financial assistance to cover health care costs, resources are available, including Government-sponsored programs and services supported by voluntary organizations.

Cancer patients and their families should discuss any concerns they may have about health care costs with their physician, medical social worker, or the business office of their hospital or clinic. The organizations and resources listed below may offer financial assistance. Organizations that provide publications in Spanish or have Spanish-speaking staff have been identified.

The American Cancer Society (ACS)

This office can provide the telephone number of the local ACS office serving your area. The local ACS office may offer reimbursement for expenses related to cancer treatment including transportation, medicine, and medical supplies. The ACS also offers programs that help cancer patients, family members, and friends cope with the emotional challenges they face. Some publications are available in Spanish. Spanish-speaking staff are available.

Tel: 1-800-ACS-2345 (1-800-227-2345)

Website: http://www.cancer.org

Excerpted from "Financial Assistance for Cancer Care," Fact Sheet 8.3, National Cancer Institute (NCI), 2000.

Community Voluntary Agencies and Service Organizations

The Salvation Army, Lutheran Social Services, Jewish Social Services, Catholic Charities, and the Lions Club may offer help. These organizations are listed in your local phone directory. Some churches and synagogues may provide financial help or services to their members.

Fundraising

This is another mechanism to consider. Some patients find that friends, family, and community members are willing to contribute financially if they are aware of a difficult situation. Contact your local library for information about how to organize fundraising efforts.

General Assistance

These programs provide food, housing, prescription drugs, and other medical expenses for those who are not eligible for other programs. Funds are often limited. Information can be obtained by contacting your state or local Department of Social Services; this number is found in the local telephone directory.

Hill-Burton

This is a program through which hospitals receive construction funds from the Federal Government. Hospitals that receive Hill-Burton funds are required by law to provide some services to people who cannot afford to pay for their hospitalization. A brochure about the program is available in Spanish.

Tel: 1-800-638-0742

Website: http://www.hrsa.dhhs.gov/osp/dfcr/obtain/consfaq.htm

Income Tax Deductions

Medical costs that are not covered by insurance policies sometimes can be deducted from annual income before taxes. Examples of tax deductible expenses might include mileage for trips to and from medical appointments, out-of-pocket costs for treatment, prescription drugs or equipment, and the cost of meals during lengthy medical visits. The local Internal Revenue Service office, tax consultants, or certified public accountants can determine medical costs that are tax deductible. These telephone numbers are available in the local telephone directory.

Website: http://www.irs.ustreas.gov

The Leukemia and Lymphoma Society (LLS)

Offers information and financial aid to patients who have leukemia, non-Hodgkin's lymphoma, Hodgkin's disease, or multiple myeloma. Callers may request a booklet describing LLS's Patient Aid Program or the telephone number for their local LLS office. Some publications are available in Spanish.

Tel: 1-800-955-4572

Website: http://www.leukemia-lymphoma.org

Medicaid (Medical Assistance)

This is a jointly funded, Federal-State health insurance program for people who need financial assistance for medical expenses, is coordinated by the Health Care Financing Administration (HCFA). At a minimum, states must provide home care services to people who receive Federal income assistance such as Social Security Income and Aid to Families with Dependent Children. Medicaid coverage includes part-time nursing, home care aide services, and medical supplies and equipment. Information about coverage is available from local state welfare offices, state health departments, state social services agencies, or the state Medicaid office. Check the local telephone directory for the number to call. Information about specific state locations is also available on the HCFA Web site. Spanish-speaking staff are available in some offices.

Website: http://www.hcfa.gov/medicaid/medicaid.htm

Medicare

A Federal health insurance program also administered by HCFA. Eligible individuals include those who are 65 or older, people of any age with permanent kidney failure, and disabled people under age 65. Medicare may offer reimbursement for some home care services. Cancer patients who qualify for Medicare may also be eligible for coverage of hospice services if they are accepted into a Medicare-certified hospice program. To receive information on eligibility, explanations of coverage, and related publications, call Medicare at the number listed below or visit their Web site. Some publications are available in Spanish.

Toll Free: 1-800-MEDICARE (1-800-633-4227)

TTY (for deaf and hard of hearing callers): 1-877-486-2048

Website: http://www.medicare.gov

The Patient Advocate Foundation (PAF)

This is a national nonprofit organization that provides education, legal counseling, and referrals to cancer patients and survivors concerning managed care, insurance, financial issues, job discrimination, and debt crisis matters.

Tel: 1-800-532-5274

Website: http://www.patientadvocate.org

Patient Assistance Programs

These programs are offered by some pharmaceutical manufacturers to help pay for medications. To learn whether a specific drug might be available at reduced cost through such a program, talk with a physician or a medical social worker.

Social Security Administration (SSA)

This is the Government agency that oversees Social Security and Supplemental Security Income. A description of each of these programs follows. More information about these and other SSA programs is available by calling the toll-free number listed below. Spanish-speaking staff are available.

Tel: 1-800-772-1213

TTY (for deaf and hard of hearing callers): 1-800-325-0778

- *Social Security*

  Provides a monthly income for eligible elderly and disabled individuals. Information on eligibility, coverage, and how to apply for benefits is available from the Social Security Administration.

  Website: http://www.ssa.gov/SSA_Home.html

- *Supplemental Security Income (SSI)*

  Supplements Social Security payments for individuals who have certain income and resource levels. SSI is administered by the Social Security Administration. Information on eligibility, coverage, and how to file a claim is available from the Social Security Administration.

  Website: http://www.ssa.gov/SSA_Home.html

Transportation

There are nonprofit organizations that arrange free or reduced cost air transportation for cancer patients going to or from cancer treatment centers. Financial need is not always a requirement. To find out about these programs, talk with a medical social worker. Ground transportation services may be offered or mileage reimbursed through the local ACS or your state or local Department of Social Services.

Veterans Benefits

Eligible veterans and their dependents may receive cancer treatment at a Veterans Administration Medical Center. Treatment for service-connected conditions is provided, and treatment for other conditions may be available based on the veteran's financial need. Some publications are available in Spanish. Spanish-speaking staff are available in some offices.

Tel: 1-800-827-1000

Website: http://www.va.gov/vbs/

Chapter 37

Links to Cancer Information on the Internet

Website that Specifically Address Prostate Cancer

CaP CURE (Association for the Cure of Cancer of the Prostate)

http://www.capcure.org

The mission of CaP CURE is to find a cure for prostate cancer. CaP CURE is a nonprofit organization that provides funding for research projects to improve methods of diagnosing and treating prostate cancer. It also offers printed resources for prostate cancer survivors and their families.

Hypertext Guide to Prostate Cancer

http://www.hypertext.org

This site gives an overview of prostate cancer, with hypertext links to detailed information on more than 250 medical Web sites.

Prostate Cancer Answers

http://www.medsch.wisc.edu/pca

This is a service of the University of Wisconsin Comprehensive Cancer Center. It provides information about prostate cancer research, prevention, detection, diagnosis, and treatment.

Excerpted from "Links to Other Cancer Information Web Sites." CancerNet, National Cancer Institute (NCI), 2001.

US TOO! International, Inc.

http://www.ustoo.com

US TOO! is a prostate cancer support group organization. Goals of US TOO! are to increase awareness of prostate cancer in the community, educate men newly diagnosed with prostate cancer, offer support groups, and provide the latest information about treatment for this disease. A limited selection of Spanish-language publications is available.

Websites That Address Many Cancer Topics

American Cancer Society (ACS)

http://www.cancer.org

800-ACS-2345

This site and the free phone line provide information to patients on cancer treatment, early detection, and prevention, as well as information on a variety of services available to cancer patients and their families.

Cancer 411

http://www.cancer411.com

Cancer 411.org came about through the efforts of The Rory Foundation and The Joyce Foundation. It seeks to help cancer patients, their families, and doctors get information through its search tools for clinical trials and organizations and its other resources.

CancerEducation.com

http://www.cancereducation.com

This site gives oncology professionals and their patients access to the latest advances in approximately 30 types of cancer, from prevention strategies and diagnostic procedures to new treatment options and advice on coping with cancer.

cancerfacts.com

http://www.cancerfacts.com

The consumer portion of the site includes interactive tools that match an individual's medical history and test results with the medical literature and generate personalized reports of treatment options, side effects, and outcomes. The consumer portion also includes email discussion groups and a list of support groups. The physician portion includes cancer literature, drug and clinical trials information, news, and online discussion forums.

Cancerpage.com

http://www.cancerpage.com

This site has news and general information, including stage-specific treatment guidelines, support chat rooms, message boards, and email access to oncology nurses covering 46 cancer information areas.

Cancer Patient Education Network (CPEN)

http://cpen.nci.nih.gov

NCI-sponsored CPEN is an organization of cancer patient education leaders from NCI-designated comprehensive and clinical centers nationwide. CPEN offers cancer patient educators and health professionals a variety of program planning and educational resources to use or to share with colleagues or patients.

CancerSource.com

http://www.cancersource.com

CancerSource.com offers disease and treatment information in a personalized and tailored manner to consumers and health professionals. Drug information, news, feature articles, community features, and relevant resources are included.

CancerTrack

http://www.cancertrack.com

CancerTrack is a source of cancer news that is updated every 15 minutes. It also gives information on books and links for many types of cancer.

Cancer Trials Support Unit

http://www.ctsu.org

The Cancer Trials Support Unit is a National Cancer Institute (NCI)-funded pilot project to facilitate participation, by both patients and physicians, in phase III NCI-sponsored cancer treatment trials.

Healthfinder

http://www.healthfinder.gov

The US Department of Health and Human Services' Healthfinder is a free gateway to reliable consumer health information. It links to online publications, clearinghouses, databases, Web sites, and support and self-help groups, as well as to government agencies and not-for-profit organizations that produce reliable information for the public.

National Foundation for Cancer Research (NFCR)

http://www.nfcr.org/html/homepage/index.html

NFCR's Web site provides information about prevention, detection, and treatment of cancers, as well as content on research for a cancer cure.

OncoLink

http://oncolink.upenn.edu

OncoLink, from the University of Pennsylvania Cancer Center, presents cancer information for patients and health care professionals. It also links to more than 50 journal and newsletter Web sites.

Oncology.com

http://www.oncology.com

Oncology.com offers information to cancer patients, families, and health care professionals. It includes disease summaries, news stories, events, and discussions on most major cancers.

Oncology Tools

http://www.fda.gov/cder/cancer

This site contains information from the FDA on cancer and approved cancer drugs. It includes summaries on different types of cancer, regulatory information, and other cancer-related resources.

Steve Dunn's CancerGuide

http://www.cancerguide.org

Maintained through the efforts of a cancer survivor, CancerGuide has links to a variety of cancer information resources and offers advice about using the information retrieved.

Sustaining Oncology Studies (SOS) Europe

http://sos.unige.it/soseuro.html

This Web site has information on support, training, and research in cancer and includes links to international meetings, cancer-related publications, and international associations.

TeleSCAN: Telematic Services in Cancer

http://telescan.nki.nl

This site contains European cancer research information for patients, health care professionals, and researchers.

Bone Marrow Transplantation

BMTInformation

http://www.bmtinfo.org/home.htm

This site provides information and data from experts in bone marrow transplantation.

BMT Support Online

http://www.bmtsupport.org

BMT Support Online is an interactive nonprofit organization that seeks to motivate, empower, and enlighten people with an interest in bone marrow transplantation through peer support and education.

National Bone Marrow Transplant Link

http://comnet.org/nbmtlink

This organization seeks to help patients and families of those considering bone marrow transplants.

National Marrow Donor Program

http://www.marrow.org

The National Marrow Donor Program, funded by the federal government, was created to improve the effectiveness of the search for bone marrow donors. It has a registry of potential bone marrow donors and provides free information on bone marrow transplantation, peripheral blood stem cell transplantation, and unrelated-donor stem cell transplantation including the use of umbilical cord blood.

Clinical Treatment Guidelines

Cancer Care Ontario Practice Guidelines Initiative

http://hiru.mcmaster.ca/ccopgi

This Web site contains clinical oncology practice guidelines produced with the support of both Cancer Care Ontario and the Ontario Ministry of Health and Long-Term Care.

Clinical Practice Guidelines

http://www.ahrq.gov/clinic/cpgsix.htm

This section of the Web site for the Agency for Healthcare Research and Quality (AHRQ) offers agency-supported clinical practice guidelines as well as guidelines on other topics.

National Guideline Clearinghouse

http://www.guideline.gov/asp/splash2.asp?cp=t&ck=t

This site contains evidence-based clinical practice guidelines. It is sponsored by the Agency for Healthcare Research and Quality (AHRQ) in partnership with the American Medical Association and the American Association of Health Plans.

Treatment Centers

HospitalWeb

http://neuro-www.mgh.harvard.edu/hospitalweb.shtml

This site has a growing collection of links to US and international hospital Web servers.

List of NCI-Designated Cancer Centers
from the NCI's Cancer Centers Program

http://www.nci.nih.gov/cancercenters/centerslist.html

The Cancer Centers Program supports research-oriented US institutions characterized by scientific excellence and their ability to integrate and focus a diversity of research approaches on the cancer problem. Three types of cancer centers are supported, based on the degree of specialization of their research approaches. The generic "cancer centers" have very focused research approaches (e.g., basic research, epidemiology research); the "clinical cancer centers" usually integrate strong basic science with strong clinical science (i.e., patient-oriented research); and the "comprehensive cancer centers" integrate strong basic, clinical, and prevention, control, and population sciences.

Prevention

American Institute for Cancer Research (AICR)

http://www.aicr.org

AICR provides information about cancer prevention, particularly through diet and nutrition. It offers a toll-free nutrition hotline, a pen pal support network, funding of research grants, and brochures and health aids about diet and nutrition and its link to cancer and cancer prevention. AICR also offers CancerResource, an information and resource program for patients. A limited selection of Spanish-language publications is available.

Cancer Research Foundation of America

http://www.preventcancer.org

The Cancer Research Foundation of America seeks to prevent cancer by funding research. The foundation also provides educational materials on early detection and nutrition.

Harvard Center for Cancer Prevention

http://www.hsph.harvard.edu/cancer

This site is designed to educate the public about cancer prevention. It includes a tool for estimating a person's cancer risk, a newsletter, and recent reports.

NCI's 5 A Day for Better Health Program

http://5aday.gov

This site includes health information, recipes, and an assessment tool for diet and physical activity.

Tobacco-Related Disease Research Program

http://www.ucop.edu/srphome/trdrp/welcome.html

This program supports innovative and creative research to reduce the human and economic cost of tobacco-related diseases.

Coping with Cancer: Specific Symptoms/Side Effects

CancerFatigue

http://www.cancerfatigue.org

This site provides tips and background information about fatigue caused by cancer and its treatment. Cancer patients and caregivers can submit personal questions about cancer fatigue and receive answers, by email, from oncology nurses.

Lymphatic Research Foundation

http://www.lymphaticresearch.org

This Web site promotes and supports biomedical research for primary and secondary lymphedemas and their associated angiodysplastic disorders.

National Lymphedema Network (NLN)

http://www.lymphnet.org

NLN provides education and guidance to lymphedema patients, health care professionals, and the public by disseminating information on the prevention and management of primary and secondary lymphedema. It has a toll-free support hotline, a referral service to treatment centers and health care professionals, a newsletter, support groups, pen pals, educational courses, and a computer database. Some Spanish-language materials are available.

Hospice Care

Hospice Education Institute

http://www.hospiceworld.org

This nonprofit organization helps patients and their families find support services in their communities. It offers information about hospice and pain management and can refer cancer patients and their families to local hospice programs.

Hospice Web

http://www.hospiceweb.com

Hospice Web stresses whole-person care and provides a means for locating suitable hospices.

314

National Hospice and Palliative Care Organization

http://www.nhpco.org

The NHPCO is an association of programs that provide hospice and palliative care. It is designed to increase awareness about hospice services and to champion the rights and issues of terminally ill patients and their families. It offers discussion groups, publications, information on how to find a hospice, and information about the financial aspects of hospice. Some Spanish-language publications are available, and staff can answer calls in Spanish.

Other Support Services

Association of Cancer Online Resources

http://www.acor.org/index.html

This site gives access to more than 75 electronic mailing lists that are designed to be public online support groups for patients, caregivers, or anyone looking for answers about cancer and related disorders.

Cancer Care

http://www.cancercare.org

Cancer Care is an organization that provides assistance free of charge to people with cancer. Its Web site has information on support services, financial assistance, and cancer treatment.

Cancer Hope Network

http://www.cancerhopenetwork.org

The trained volunteers of this not-for-profit organization provide free, one-on-one support to cancer patients and their families.

Cancer Supportive Care Program

http://www.cancersupportivecare.com

This site contains a range of supportive care information. Topics include nutrition, fatigue, anemia, pain control, and lymphedema.

Corporate Angel Network

http://www.corpangelnetwork.org

The Corporate Angel Network (CAN) provides cancer patients with free air transportation to and from recognized treatment centers in the United States. CAN uses empty seats on corporate aircraft operating on business flights. Patients must meet CAN's qualifications but do not need to meet any financial-need criteria.

Gilda's Club, Inc.

http://www.gildasclub.org

Gilda's Club provides social and emotional support to cancer patients, their families, and friends. Lectures, workshops, networking groups, special events, and a children's program are available.

Make-A-Wish Foundation

http://www.wish.org

This charitable organization serves as a resource for those who may know of a child with a life-threatening illness that may qualify for a wish.

Patient Advocate Foundation (PAF)

http://www.patientadvocate.org

PAF provides education, legal counseling, and referrals to cancer patients and survivors concerning managed care, insurance, financial issues, job discrimination, and debt crisis matters.

R.A. Bloch Cancer Foundation, Inc.

http://www.blochcancer.org

This site is designed for newly diagnosed cancer patients. The focus of the foundation is to help all cancer patients conquer their disease.

STARBRIGHT Foundation

http://www.starbright.org

This foundation creates projects to help seriously ill children and adolescents cope with the challenges they face. It produces materials such as interactive educational CD-ROMs and videos about medical conditions and procedures, gives advice on talking with a health professional, and covers other issues related to children and adolescents with serious medical conditions. All materials are available free of charge. Staff can respond to calls in Spanish.

Vital Options and "The Group Room" Cancer Radio Talk Show

http://www.vitaloptions.org

The mission of Vital Options is to use communications technology to reach people dealing with cancer. This organization holds a weekly syndicated call-in cancer talk show linking callers with other patients, long-term survivors, family members, physicians, and therapists experienced in working with and discussing cancer issues.

The Wellness Community

http://www.wellness-community.org

The Wellness Community gives free psychological and emotional support to cancer patients and their families. It offers support groups facilitated by licensed therapists, stress reduction and cancer education workshops, nutrition guidance, exercise sessions, and social events.

Cancer Literature

American Association for Cancer Research (AACR)

http://www.aacr.org

This Web site allows users to search for information in AACR journals and in annual meeting abstracts.

American Society of Clinical Oncology (ASCO)

http://www.asco.org

This site allows users to search the Journal of Clinical Oncology and the ASCO annual meeting abstracts.

Cancer News on the Net

http://www.cancernews.com

Cancer News on the Net features original articles about many types of cancer. It also links to other sites that contain cancer information.

Electronic Journal of Oncology

http://ejo.univ-lyon1.fr

This exclusively online journal contains peer-reviewed original publications in the fields of oncology and neoplastic hematology.

Internet Grateful Med

http://igm.nlm.nih.gov

Internet Grateful Med provides free access to MEDLINE, AIDSLINE, BIOETHICSLINE, ChemID, TOXLINE, and other National Library of Medicine databases. It also has links to PubMed (MEDLINE and PREMEDLINE) and MEDLINEplus for consumer health information.

MEDLINE Journals With Links to Publisher Web Sites

http://www.ncbi.nlm.nih.gov/PubMed/fulltext.html

This site lists hundreds of journals in MEDLINE for which publishers have provided links to their journal Web sites.

MEDLINEplus

http://www.nlm.nih.gov/medlineplus/cancers.html

This Web site offers information and medical literature from the National Library of Medicine and has numerous links to other sites.

NCI Publications Locator

http://cissecure.nci.nih.gov/ncipubs

This site accesses National Cancer Institute publications. It allows Web users to order printed materials to be mailed to them and also links NCI materials that may be viewed and downloaded from the Web.

SOS Europe's Cancer Related Publications On Line

http://sos.unige.it/soseuro/oncopubl/titles.html

A service of the Sustaining Oncology Studies Europe Information Resource (SOS Europe), this site contains links to more than 200 journal Web sites.

Cancer Statistics

American Cancer Society Statistics

http://www3.cancer.org/cancerinfo/
sitecenter.asp?ctid=8&scp=0&scs=0&scss=0&scdoc=40000

The American Cancer Society tracks cancer occurrence, including the number of deaths and cases, and how long people survive after diagnosis.

CDC's National Program of Cancer Registries (NPCR)

http://www.cdc.gov/cancer/npcr

Established by Congress in 1992, NPCR supports efforts by states and territories of the United States to initiate and improve cancer registries and to establish a computerized reporting and data-processing system.

Surveillance, Epidemiology, and End Results (SEER)

http://www-seer.ims.nci.nih.gov

The SEER program of the National Cancer Institute collects and publishes cancer incidence and survival data from population-based cancer registries that include approximately 14 percent of the US population.

Other Resources

Minority Health

Intercultural Cancer Council

http://icc.bcm.tmc.edu/home.htm

This Web site is designed to serve the minority and medically underserved communities by providing cancer-related information.

Office of Minority Health

http://www.omhrc.gov

This site contains information on a variety of subjects that affect the health of racial and ethnic populations, including cancer.

Information in Spanish

Cancer Care

http://www.cancercare.org

Cancer Care is an organization that provides assistance free of charge to people with cancer. Its Web site has information on support services, financial assistance, and cancer treatment.

NOAH: New York Online Access to Health

http://www.noah-health.org/index.html

This site offers a wide selection of cancer information. Much of it is available in Spanish and English.

Complementary/Alternative Medicine

National Center for Complementary and Alternative Medicine (NCCAM)

http://nccam.nih.gov

NCCAM facilitates and supports basic and applied research of complementary and alternative medicine (CAM) modalities. It sponsors training for researchers and disseminates information about CAM therapies to practitioners and to the public.

Office of Cancer Complementary and Alternative Medicine (OCCAM)

http://occam.nci.nih.gov

OCCAM supports and facilitates the development of NCI-supported complementary and alternative medicine (CAM) cancer research, coordinates NCI's collaborations with the National Center for Complementary and Alternative Medicine, and provides an interface for the NCI with the public, health practitioners, and researchers regarding CAM cancer issues.

Associations and Societies

American Association for Cancer Research (AACR)

http://www.aacr.org

This site contains information on AACR membership, meetings, journals, and conferences.

American Society of Clinical Oncology (ASCO)

http://www.asco.org

This site has cancer information for patients, including information on treatment, support groups, and other resources. The information for health professionals includes ASCO policies, meetings, and publications.

Association of Community Cancer Centers (ACCC)

http://www.accc-cancer.org

This Web site features in-depth profiles of ACCC member hospital cancer programs, legislative updates, reimbursement information, standards for cancer programs, and patient-management guidelines.

National Coalition for Cancer Survivorship (NCCS)

http://www.cansearch.org

NCCS is a network of groups and individuals that provide information and resources on cancer advocacy, support, and quality-of-life issues. A section of the Web site and a limited selection of publications are available in Spanish.

ONS Online

http://www.ons.org

ONS Online is an information service of the Oncology Nursing Society (ONS). It offers information about the organization and its programs and products, as well as news, ONS publications, and links to other cancer-related sites.

Society of Surgical Oncology

http://www.surgonc.org

This site contains information on practice guidelines, training programs, meetings, abstracts, and publications to promote optimal standards for the multimodal care of surgical patients with cancer.

US Government Websites

Agency for Healthcare Research and Quality (AHRQ)

http://www.ahrq.gov

This site contains information from the offices and centers of the AHRQ, including news, resources, information for consumers, and a catalog of information products.

Centers for Disease Control and Prevention (CDC)

http://www.cdc.gov

The CDC Web site provides publications, travelers' health information, statistics, and training, employment, and other information.

Food and Drug Administration (FDA)

http://www.fda.gov

This site contains information about the FDA, including information on medical devices, biologics, drugs, and drug regulation.

National Center for Biotechnology Information

http://www.ncbi.nlm.nih.gov

This site, for a division of the National Library of Medicine (NLM), includes GenBank, the National Institutes of Health genetic sequence database, as well as other sources of biomedical information.

National Institute of Environmental Health Sciences (NIEHS)

http://www.niehs.nih.gov

NIEHS, one of the institutes of NIH, studies human health and disease as they relate to environmental factors, individual susceptibility, and age.

National Institutes of Health (NIH)

http://www.nih.gov

NIH is a component of the US Department of Health and Human Services. It consists of 25 institutes and centers that conduct medical research for the federal government.

National Toxicology Program (NTP)

http://ntp-server.niehs.nih.gov

NTP, an agency of the Department of Health and Human Services, provides information about potentially toxic chemicals to regulatory and research agencies and to the public.

National Women's Health Information Center (NWHIC)

http://www.4women.gov

This Web site is sponsored by the Office on Women's Health in the Department of Health and Human Services. It provides a broad array of reliable, commercial-free health publications and referrals to health-related organizations for women. Some of this information is available in Spanish.

The White House

http://www.whitehouse.gov

The White House Web site links to all other US government sites.

Index

Index

325

Health Reference Series
COMPLETE CATALOG

AIDS Sourcebook, 1st Edition

Basic Information about AIDS and HIV Infection, Featuring Historical and Statistical Data, Current Research, Prevention, and Other Special Topics of Interest for Persons Living with AIDS

Along with Source Listings for Further Assistance

Edited by Karen Bellenir and Peter D. Dresser. 831 pages. 1995. 0-7808-0031-1. $78.

"One strength of this book is its practical emphasis. The intended audience is the lay reader ... useful as an educational tool for health care providers who work with AIDS patients. Recommended for public libraries as well as hospital or academic libraries that collect consumer materials."
— *Bulletin of the Medical Library Association, Jan '96*

"This is the most comprehensive volume of its kind on an important medical topic. Highly recommended for all libraries."
— *Reference Book Review, '96*

"Very useful reference for all libraries."
— *Choice, Association of College and Research Libraries, Oct '95*

"There is a wealth of information here that can provide much educational assistance. It is a must book for all libraries and should be on the desk of each and every congressional leader. Highly recommended."
— *AIDS Book Review Journal, Aug '95*

"Recommended for most collections."
— *Library Journal, Jul '95*

■

AIDS Sourcebook, 2nd Edition

Basic Consumer Health Information about Acquired Immune Deficiency Syndrome (AIDS) and Human Immunodeficiency Virus (HIV) Infection, Featuring Updated Statistical Data, Reports on Recent Research and Prevention Initiatives, and Other Special Topics of Interest for Persons Living with AIDS, Including New Antiretroviral Treatment Options, Strategies for Combating Opportunistic Infections, Information about Clinical Trials, and More

Along with a Glossary of Important Terms and Resource Listings for Further Help and Information

Edited by Karen Bellenir. 751 pages. 1999. 0-7808-0225-X. $78.

"Highly recommended."
— *American Reference Books Annual, 2000*

"Excellent sourcebook. This continues to be a highly recommended book. There is no other book that provides as much information as this book provides."
— *AIDS Book Review Journal, Dec-Jan 2000*

"Recommended reference source."
— *Booklist, American Library Association, Dec '99*

"A solid text for college-level health libraries."
— *The Bookwatch, Aug '99*

Cited in *Reference Sources for Small and Medium-Sized Libraries*, American Library Association, 1999

■

Alcoholism Sourcebook

Basic Consumer Health Information about the Physical and Mental Consequences of Alcohol Abuse, Including Liver Disease, Pancreatitis, Wernicke-Korsakoff Syndrome (Alcoholic Dementia), Fetal Alcohol Syndrome, Heart Disease, Kidney Disorders, Gastrointestinal Problems, and Immune System Compromise and Featuring Facts about Addiction, Detoxification, Alcohol Withdrawal, Recovery, and the Maintenance of Sobriety

Along with a Glossary and Directories of Resources for Further Help and Information

Edited by Karen Bellenir. 613 pages. 2000. 0-7808-0325-6. $78.

"This title is one of the few reference works on alcoholism for general readers. For some readers this will be a welcome complement to the many self-help books on the market. Recommended for collections serving general readers and consumer health collections."
— *E-Streams, Mar '01*

"This book is an excellent choice for public and academic libraries."
— *American Reference Books Annual, 2001*

"Recommended reference source."
— *Booklist, American Library Association, Dec '00*

"Presents a wealth of information on alcohol use and abuse and its effects on the body and mind, treatment, and prevention."
— *SciTech Book News, Dec '00*

"Important new health guide which packs in the latest consumer information about the problems of alcoholism."
— *Reviewer's Bookwatch, Nov '00*

SEE ALSO Drug Abuse Sourcebook, Substance Abuse Sourcebook

■

Allergies Sourcebook, 1st Edition

Basic Information about Major Forms and Mechanisms of Common Allergic Reactions, Sensitivities, and Intolerances, Including Anaphylaxis, Asthma, Hives and Other Dermatologic Symptoms, Rhinitis, and Sinusitis

Along with Their Usual Triggers Like Animal Fur, Chemicals, Drugs, Dust, Foods, Insects, Latex, Pollen, and Poison Ivy, Oak, and Sumac; Plus Information on Prevention, Identification, and Treatment

Edited by Allan R. Cook. 611 pages. 1997. 0-7808-0036-2. $78.

Allergies Sourcebook, 2nd Edition

Basic Consumer Health Information about Allergic Disorders, Triggers, Reactions, and Related Symptoms, Including Anaphylaxis, Rhinitis, Sinusitis, Asthma, Dermatitis, Conjunctivitis, and Multiple Chemical Sensitivity

Along with Tips on Diagnosis, Prevention, and Treatment, Statistical Data, a Glossary, and a Directory of Sources for Further Help and Information

Edited by Annemarie S. Muth. 600 pages. 2001. 0-7808-0376-0. $78.

Alternative Medicine Sourcebook

Basic Consumer Health Information about Alternatives to Conventional Medicine, Including Acupressure, Acupuncture, Aromatherapy, Ayurveda, Bioelectromagnetics, Environmental Medicine, Essence Therapy, Food and Nutrition Therapy, Herbal Therapy, Homeopathy, Imaging, Massage, Naturopathy, Reflexology, Relaxation and Meditation, Sound Therapy, Vitamin and Mineral Therapy, and Yoga, and More

Edited by Allan R. Cook. 737 pages. 1999. 0-7808-0200-4. $78.

"Recommended reference source."
—Booklist, American Library Association, Feb '00

"A great addition to the reference collection of every type of library." —American Reference Books Annual, 2000

Alzheimer's, Stroke & 29 Other Neurological Disorders Sourcebook, 1st Edition

Basic Information for the Layperson on 31 Diseases or Disorders Affecting the Brain and Nervous System, First Describing the Illness, Then Listing Symptoms, Diagnostic Methods, and Treatment Options, and Including Statistics on Incidences and Causes

Edited by Frank E. Bair. 579 pages. 1993. 1-55888-748-2. $78.

"Nontechnical reference book that provides reader-friendly information."
—Family Caregiver Alliance Update, Winter '96

"Should be included in any library's patient education section." —American Reference Books Annual, 1994

"Written in an approachable and accessible style. Recommended for patient education and consumer health collections in health science center and public libraries." —Academic Library Book Review, Dec '93

"It is very handy to have information on more than thirty neurological disorders under one cover, and there is no recent source like it." —Reference Quarterly, American Library Association, Fall '93

SEE ALSO Brain Disorders Sourcebook

Alzheimer's Disease Sourcebook, 2nd Edition

Basic Consumer Health Information about Alzheimer's Disease, Related Disorders, and Other Dementias, Including Multi-Infarct Dementia, AIDS-Related Dementia, Alcoholic Dementia, Huntington's Disease, Delirium, and Confusional States

Along with Reports Detailing Current Research Efforts in Prevention and Treatment, Long-Term Care Issues, and Listings of Sources for Additional Help and Information

Edited by Karen Bellenir. 524 pages. 1999. 0-7808-0223-3. $78.

"Provides a wealth of useful information not otherwise available in one place. This resource is recommended for all types of libraries."
—American Reference Books Annual, 2000

"Recommended reference source."
—Booklist, American Library Association, Oct '99

Arthritis Sourcebook

Basic Consumer Health Information about Specific Forms of Arthritis and Related Disorders, Including Rheumatoid Arthritis, Osteoarthritis, Gout, Polymyalgia Rheumatica, Psoriatic Arthritis, Spondyloarthropathies, Juvenile Rheumatoid Arthritis, and Juvenile Ankylosing Spondylitis

Along with Information about Medical, Surgical, and Alternative Treatment Options, and Including Strategies for Coping with Pain, Fatigue, and Stress

Edited by Allan R. Cook. 550 pages. 1998. 0-7808-0201-2. $78.

"... accessible to the layperson."
—Reference and Research Book News, Feb '99

Asthma Sourcebook

Basic Consumer Health Information about Asthma, Including Symptoms, Traditional and Nontraditional Remedies, Treatment Advances, Quality-of-Life Aids, Medical Research Updates, and the Role of Allergies, Exercise, Age, the Environment, and Genetics in the Development of Asthma

Along with Statistical Data, a Glossary, and Directories of Support Groups, and Other Resources for Further Information

Edited by Annemarie S. Muth. 628 pages. 2000. 0-7808-0381-7. $78.

"A worthwhile reference acquisition for public libraries and academic medical libraries whose readers desire a quick introduction to the wide range of asthma information." —Choice, Association of College and Research Libraries, Jun '01

"Recommended reference source."
—Booklist, American Library Association, Feb '01

"Highly recommended." — *The Bookwatch, Jan '01*

"There is much good information for patients and their families who deal with asthma daily."
— *American Medical Writers Association Journal, Winter '01*

"This informative text is recommended for consumer health collections in public, secondary school, and community college libraries and the libraries of universities with a large undergraduate population."
— *American Reference Books Annual, 2001*

■

Back & Neck Disorders Sourcebook

Basic Information about Disorders and Injuries of the Spinal Cord and Vertebrae, Including Facts on Chiropractic Treatment, Surgical Interventions, Paralysis, and Rehabilitation

Along with Advice for Preventing Back Trouble

Edited by Karen Bellenir. 548 pages. 1997. 0-7808-0202-0. $78.

"The strength of this work is its basic, easy-to-read format. Recommended."
— *Reference and User Services Quarterly, American Library Association, Winter '97*

■

Blood & Circulatory Disorders Sourcebook

Basic Information about Blood and Its Components, Anemias, Leukemias, Bleeding Disorders, and Circulatory Disorders, Including Aplastic Anemia, Thalassemia, Sickle-Cell Disease, Hemochromatosis, Hemophilia, Von Willebrand Disease, and Vascular Diseases

Along with a Special Section on Blood Transfusions and Blood Supply Safety, a Glossary, and Source Listings for Further Help and Information

Edited by Karen Bellenir and Linda M. Shin. 554 pages. 1998. 0-7808-0203-9. $78.

"Recommended reference source."
— *Booklist, American Library Association, Feb '99*

"An important reference sourcebook written in simple language for everyday, non-technical users. "
— *Reviewer's Bookwatch, Jan '99*

■

Brain Disorders Sourcebook

Basic Consumer Health Information about Strokes, Epilepsy, Amyotrophic Lateral Sclerosis (ALS/Lou Gehrig's Disease), Parkinson's Disease, Brain Tumors, Cerebral Palsy, Headache, Tourette Syndrome, and More

Along with Statistical Data, Treatment and Rehabilitation Options, Coping Strategies, Reports on Current

Research Initiatives, a Glossary, and Resource Listings for Additional Help and Information

Edited by Karen Bellenir. 481 pages. 1999. 0-7808-0229-2. $78.

"Belongs on the shelves of any library with a consumer health collection." — *E-Streams, Mar '00*

"Recommended reference source."
— *Booklist, American Library Association, Oct '99*

SEE ALSO *Alzheimer's, Stroke & 29 Other Neurological Disorders Sourcebook, 1st Edition*

■

Breast Cancer Sourcebook

Basic Consumer Health Information about Breast Cancer, Including Diagnostic Methods, Treatment Options, Alternative Therapies, Self-Help Information, Related Health Concerns, Statistical and Demographic Data, and Facts for Men with Breast Cancer

Along with Reports on Current Research Initiatives, a Glossary of Related Medical Terms, and a Directory of Sources for Further Help and Information

Edited by Edward J. Prucha and Karen Bellenir. 580 pages. 2001. 0-7808-0244-6. $78.

SEE ALSO *Cancer Sourcebook for Women, 1st and 2nd Editions, Women's Health Concerns Sourcebook*

■

Breastfeeding Sourcebook

Basic Consumer Health Information about the Benefits of Breastmilk, Preparing to Breastfeed, Breastfeeding as a Baby Grows, Nutrition, and More, Including Information on Special Situations and Concerns, Such as Mastitis, Illness, Medications, Allergies, Multiple Births, Prematurity, Special Needs, and Adoption

Along with a Glossary and Resources for Additional Help and Information

Edited by Jenni Lynn Colson. 350 pages. 2001. 0-7808-0332-9. $48.

SEE ALSO *Pregnancy & Birth Sourcebook*

■

Burns Sourcebook

Basic Consumer Health Information about Various Types of Burns and Scalds, Including Flame, Heat, Cold, Electrical, Chemical, and Sun Burns

Along with Information on Short-Term and Long-Term Treatments, Tissue Reconstruction, Plastic Surgery, Prevention Suggestions, and First Aid

Edited by Allan R. Cook. 604 pages. 1999. 0-7808-0204-7. $78.

"This key reference guide is an invaluable addition to all health care and public libraries in confronting this ongoing health issue."
— *American Reference Books Annual, 2000*

"This is an exceptional addition to the series and is highly recommended for all consumer health collections, hospital libraries, and academic medical centers." — *E-Streams, Mar '00*

"Recommended reference source." — *Booklist, American Library Association, Dec '99*

SEE ALSO Skin Disorders Sourcebook

■

Cancer Sourcebook, 1st Edition

Basic Information on Cancer Types, Symptoms, Diagnostic Methods, and Treatments, Including Statistics on Cancer Occurrences Worldwide and the Risks Associated with Known Carcinogens and Activities

Edited by Frank E. Bair. 932 pages. 1990. 1-55888-888-8. $78.

Cited in *Reference Sources for Small and Medium-Sized Libraries*, American Library Association, 1999

"Written in nontechnical language. Useful for patients, their families, medical professionals, and librarians." — *Guide to Reference Books, 1996*

"Designed with the non-medical professional in mind. Libraries and medical facilities interested in patient education should certainly consider adding the *Cancer Sourcebook* to their holdings. This compact collection of reliable information . . . is an invaluable tool for helping patients and patients' families and friends to take the first steps in coping with the many difficulties of cancer." — *Medical Reference Services Quarterly, Winter '91*

"Specifically created for the nontechnical reader . . . an important resource for the general reader trying to understand the complexities of cancer." — *American Reference Books Annual, 1991*

"This publication's nontechnical nature and very comprehensive format make it useful for both the general public and undergraduate students." — *Choice, Association of College and Research Libraries, Oct '90*

■

New Cancer Sourcebook, 2nd Edition

Basic Information about Major Forms and Stages of Cancer, Featuring Facts about Primary and Secondary Tumors of the Respiratory, Nervous, Lymphatic, Circulatory, Skeletal, and Gastrointestinal Systems, and Specific Organs; Statistical and Demographic Data; Treatment Options; and Strategies for Coping

Edited by Allan R. Cook. 1,313 pages. 1996. 0-7808-0041-9. $78.

"An excellent resource for patients with newly diagnosed cancer and their families. The dialogue is simple, direct, and comprehensive. Highly recommended for patients and families to aid in their understanding of cancer and its treatment." — *Booklist Health Sciences Supplement, American Library Association, Oct '97*

"The amount of factual and useful information is extensive. The writing is very clear, geared to general readers. Recommended for all levels." — *Choice, Association of College and Research Libraries, Jan '97*

■

Cancer Sourcebook, 3rd Edition

Basic Consumer Health Information about Major Forms and Stages of Cancer, Featuring Facts about Primary and Secondary Tumors of the Respiratory, Nervous, Lymphatic, Circulatory, Skeletal, and Gastrointestinal Systems, and Specific Organs

Along with Statistical and Demographic Data, Treatment Options, Strategies for Coping, a Glossary, and a Directory of Sources for Additional Help and Information

Edited by Edward J. Prucha. 1,069 pages. 2000. 0-7808-0227-6. $78.

"This title is recommended for health sciences and public libraries with consumer health collections." — *E-Streams, Feb '01*

". . . can be effectively used by cancer patients and their families who are looking for answers in a language they can understand. Public and hospital libraries should have it on their shelves." — *American Reference Books Annual, 2001*

"Recommended reference source." — *Booklist, American Library Association, Dec '00*

■

Cancer Sourcebook for Women, 1st Edition

Basic Information about Specific Forms of Cancer That Affect Women, Featuring Facts about Breast Cancer, Cervical Cancer, Ovarian Cancer, Cancer of the Uterus and Uterine Sarcoma, Cancer of the Vagina, and Cancer of the Vulva; Statistical and Demographic Data; Treatments, Self-Help Management Suggestions, and Current Research Initiatives

Edited by Allan R. Cook and Peter D. Dresser. 524 pages. 1996. 0-7808-0076-1. $78.

". . . written in easily understandable, non-technical language. Recommended for public libraries or hospital and academic libraries that collect patient education or consumer health materials." — *Medical Reference Services Quarterly, Spring '97*

"Would be of value in a consumer health library. . . . written with the health care consumer in mind. Medical jargon is at a minimum, and medical terms are explained in clear, understandable sentences." — *Bulletin of the Medical Library Association, Oct '96*

"The availability under one cover of all these pertinent publications, grouped under cohesive headings, makes this certainly a most useful sourcebook." — *Choice, Association of College and Research Libraries, Jun '96*

"Presents a comprehensive knowledge base for general readers. Men and women both benefit from the gold mine of information nestled between the two covers of this book. Recommended."
—*Academic Library Book Review, Summer '96*

"This timely book is highly recommended for consumer health and patient education collections in all libraries." — *Library Journal, Apr '96*

SEE ALSO *Breast Cancer Sourcebook, Women's Health Concerns Sourcebook*

■

Cancer Sourcebook for Women, 2nd Edition

Basic Consumer Health Information about Specific Forms of Cancer That Affect Women, Including Cervical Cancer, Ovarian Cancer, Endometrial Cancer, Uterine Sarcoma, Vaginal Cancer, Vulvar Cancer, and Gestational Trophoblastic Tumor; and Featuring Statistical Information, Facts about Tests and Treatments, a Glossary of Cancer Terms, and an Extensive List of Additional Resources

Edited by Karen Bellenir. 600 pages. 2001. 0-7808-0226-8. $78.

SEE ALSO *Breast Cancer Sourcebook, Women's Health Concerns Sourcebook*

■

Cardiovascular Diseases & Disorders Sourcebook, 1st Edition

Basic Information about Cardiovascular Diseases and Disorders, Featuring Facts about the Cardiovascular System, Demographic and Statistical Data, Descriptions of Pharmacological and Surgical Interventions, Lifestyle Modifications, and a Special Section Focusing on Heart Disorders in Children

Edited by Karen Bellenir and Peter D. Dresser. 683 pages. 1995. 0-7808-0032-X. $78.

". . . comprehensive format provides an extensive overview on this subject."
—*Choice, Association of College and Research Libraries, Jun '96*

". . . an easily understood, complete, up-to-date resource. This well executed public health tool will make valuable information available to those that need it most, patients and their families. The typeface, sturdy non-reflective paper, and library binding add a feel of quality found wanting in other publications. Highly recommended for academic and general libraries. "
—*Academic Library Book Review, Summer '96*

SEE ALSO *Healthy Heart Sourcebook for Women, Heart Diseases & Disorders Sourcebook, 2nd Edition*

Caregiving Sourcebook

Basic Consumer Health Information for Caregivers, Including a Profile of Caregivers, Caregiving Responsibilities and Concerns, Tips for Specific Conditions, Care Environments, and the Effects of Caregiving

Along with Facts about Legal Issues, Financial Information, and Future Planning, a Glossary, and a Listing of Additional Resources

Edited by Joyce Brennfleck Shannon. 600 pages. 2001. 0-7808-0331-0. $78.

■

Colds, Flu & Other Common Ailments Sourcebook

Basic Consumer Health Information about Common Ailments and Injuries, Including Colds, Coughs, the Flu, Sinus Problems, Headaches, Fever, Nausea and Vomiting, Menstrual Cramps, Diarrhea, Constipation, Hemorrhoids, Back Pain, Dandruff, Dry and Itchy Skin, Cuts, Scrapes, Sprains, Bruises, and More

Along with Information about Prevention, Self-Care, Choosing a Doctor, Over-the-Counter Medications, Folk Remedies, and Alternative Therapies, and Including a Glossary of Important Terms and a Directory of Resources for Further Help and Information

Edited by Chad T. Kimball. 638 pages. 2001. 0-7808-0435-X. $78.

■

Communication Disorders Sourcebook

Basic Information about Deafness and Hearing Loss, Speech and Language Disorders, Voice Disorders, Balance and Vestibular Disorders, and Disorders of Smell, Taste, and Touch

Edited by Linda M. Ross. 533 pages. 1996. 0-7808-0077-X. $78.

"This is skillfully edited and is a welcome resource for the layperson. It should be found in every public and medical library." — *Booklist Health Sciences Supplement, American Library Association, Oct '97*

■

Congenital Disorders Sourcebook

Basic Information about Disorders Acquired during Gestation, Including Spina Bifida, Hydrocephalus, Cerebral Palsy, Heart Defects, Craniofacial Abnormalities, Fetal Alcohol Syndrome, and More

Along with Current Treatment Options and Statistical Data

Edited by Karen Bellenir. 607 pages. 1997. 0-7808-0205-5. $78.

"Recommended reference source."
— *Booklist, American Library Association, Oct '97*

SEE ALSO *Pregnancy & Birth Sourcebook*

Consumer Issues in Health Care Sourcebook

Basic Information about Health Care Fundamentals and Related Consumer Issues, Including Exams and Screening Tests, Physician Specialties, Choosing a Doctor, Using Prescription and Over-the-Counter Medications Safely, Avoiding Health Scams, Managing Common Health Risks in the Home, Care Options for Chronically or Terminally Ill Patients, and a List of Resources for Obtaining Help and Further Information

Edited by Karen Bellenir. 618 pages. 1998. 0-7808-0221-7. $78.

"Both public and academic libraries will want to have a copy in their collection for readers who are interested in self-education on health issues."
—American Reference Books Annual, 2000

"The editor has researched the literature from government agencies and others, saving readers the time and effort of having to do the research themselves. Recommended for public libraries."
—Reference and User Services Quarterly, American Library Association, Spring '99

"Recommended reference source."
—Booklist, American Library Association, Dec '98

■

Contagious & Non-Contagious Infectious Diseases Sourcebook

Basic Information about Contagious Diseases like Measles, Polio, Hepatitis B, and Infectious Mononucleosis, and Non-Contagious Infectious Diseases like Tetanus and Toxic Shock Syndrome, and Diseases Occurring as Secondary Infections Such as Shingles and Reye Syndrome

Along with Vaccination, Prevention, and Treatment Information, and a Section Describing Emerging Infectious Disease Threats

Edited by Karen Bellenir and Peter D. Dresser. 566 pages. 1996. 0-7808-0075-3. $78.

■

Death & Dying Sourcebook

Basic Consumer Health Information for the Layperson about End-of-Life Care and Related Ethical and Legal Issues, Including Chief Causes of Death, Autopsies, Pain Management for the Terminally Ill, Life Support Systems, Insurance, Euthanasia, Assisted Suicide, Hospice Programs, Living Wills, Funeral Planning, Counseling, Mourning, Organ Donation, and Physician Training

Along with Statistical Data, a Glossary, and Listings of Sources for Further Help and Information

Edited by Annemarie S. Muth. 641 pages. 1999. 0-7808-0230-6. $78.

"Public libraries, medical libraries, and academic libraries will all find this sourcebook a useful addition to their collections."
—American Reference Books Annual, 2001

"An extremely useful resource for those concerned with death and dying in the United States."
—Respiratory Care, Nov '00

"Recommended reference source."
—Booklist, American Library Association, Aug '00

"This book is a definite must for all those involved in end-of-life care."
—Doody's Review Service, 2000

■

Diabetes Sourcebook, 1st Edition

Basic Information about Insulin-Dependent and Non-insulin-Dependent Diabetes Mellitus, Gestational Diabetes, and Diabetic Complications, Symptoms, Treatment, and Research Results, Including Statistics on Prevalence, Morbidity, and Mortality

Along with Source Listings for Further Help and Information

Edited by Karen Bellenir and Peter D. Dresser. 827 pages. 1994. 1-55888-751-2. $78.

". . . very informative and understandable for the layperson without being simplistic. It provides a comprehensive overview for laypersons who want a general understanding of the disease or who want to focus on various aspects of the disease."
—Bulletin of the Medical Library Association, Jan '96

■

Diabetes Sourcebook, 2nd Edition

Basic Consumer Health Information about Type 1 Diabetes (Insulin-Dependent or Juvenile-Onset Diabetes), Type 2 (Noninsulin-Dependent or Adult-Onset Diabetes), Gestational Diabetes, and Related Disorders, Including Diabetes Prevalence Data, Management Issues, the Role of Diet and Exercise in Controlling Diabetes, Insulin and Other Diabetes Medicines, and Complications of Diabetes Such as Eye Diseases, Periodontal Disease, Amputation, and End-Stage Renal Disease

Along with Reports on Current Research Initiatives, a Glossary, and Resource Listings for Further Help and Information

Edited by Karen Bellenir. 688 pages. 1998. 0-7808-0224-1. $78.

"This comprehensive book is an excellent addition for high school, academic, medical, and public libraries. This volume is highly recommended."
—American Reference Books Annual, 2000

"An invaluable reference." —Library Journal, May '00

Selected as one of the 250 "Best Health Sciences Books of 1999." —Doody's Rating Service, Mar-Apr 2000

"Recommended reference source."
—Booklist, American Library Association, Feb '99

". . . provides reliable mainstream medical information . . . belongs on the shelves of any library with a consumer health collection." —E-Streams, Sep '99

"Provides useful information for the general public."
—Healthlines, University of Michigan Health Management Research Center, Sep/Oct '99

Diet & Nutrition Sourcebook, 1st Edition

Basic Information about Nutrition, Including the Dietary Guidelines for Americans, the Food Guide Pyramid, and Their Applications in Daily Diet, Nutritional Advice for Specific Age Groups, Current Nutritional Issues and Controversies, the New Food Label and How to Use It to Promote Healthy Eating, and Recent Developments in Nutritional Research

Edited by Dan R. Harris. 662 pages. 1996. 0-7808-0084-2. $78.

"Useful reference as a food and nutrition sourcebook for the general consumer." — *Booklist Health Sciences Supplement, American Library Association, Oct '97*

"Recommended for public libraries and medical libraries that receive general information requests on nutrition. It is readable and will appeal to those interested in learning more about healthy dietary practices." — *Medical Reference Services Quarterly, Fall '97*

"An abundance of medical and social statistics is translated into readable information geared toward the general reader." — *Bookwatch, Mar '97*

"With dozens of questionable diet books on the market, it is so refreshing to find a reliable and factual reference book. Recommended to aspiring professionals, librarians, and others seeking and giving reliable dietary advice. An excellent compilation." — *Choice, Association of College and Research Libraries, Feb '97*

SEE ALSO *Digestive Diseases & Disorders Sourcebook, Gastrointestinal Diseases & Disorders Sourcebook*

Diet & Nutrition Sourcebook, 2nd Edition

Basic Consumer Health Information about Dietary Guidelines, Recommended Daily Intake Values, Vitamins, Minerals, Fiber, Fat, Weight Control, Dietary Supplements, and Food Additives

Along with Special Sections on Nutrition Needs throughout Life and Nutrition for People with Such Specific Medical Concerns as Allergies, High Blood Cholesterol, Hypertension, Diabetes, Celiac Disease, Seizure Disorders, Phenylketonuria (PKU), Cancer, and Eating Disorders, and Including Reports on Current Nutrition Research and Source Listings for Additional Help and Information

Edited by Karen Bellenir. 650 pages. 1999. 0-7808-0228-4. $78.

"This book is an excellent source of basic diet and nutrition information." — *Booklist Health Sciences Supplement, American Library Association, Dec '00*

"This reference document should be in any public library, but it would be a very good guide for beginning students in the health sciences. If the other books in this publisher's series are as good as this, they should all be in the health sciences collections." — *American Reference Books Annual, 2000*

"This book is an excellent general nutrition reference for consumers who desire to take an active role in their health care for prevention. Consumers of all ages who select this book can feel confident that they are receiving current and accurate information." — *Journal of Nutrition for the Elderly, Vol. 19, No. 4, '00*

"Recommended reference source." — *Booklist, American Library Association, Dec '99*

SEE ALSO *Digestive Diseases & Disorders Sourcebook, Gastrointestinal Diseases & Disorders Sourcebook*

Digestive Diseases & Disorders Sourcebook

Basic Consumer Health Information about Diseases and Disorders that Impact the Upper and Lower Digestive System, Including Celiac Disease, Constipation, Crohn's Disease, Cyclic Vomiting Syndrome, Diarrhea, Diverticulosis and Diverticulitis, Gallstones, Heartburn, Hemorrhoids, Hernias, Indigestion (Dyspepsia), Irritable Bowel Syndrome, Lactose Intolerance, Ulcers, and More

Along with Information about Medications and Other Treatments, Tips for Maintaining a Healthy Digestive Tract, a Glossary, and Directory of Digestive Diseases Organizations

Edited by Karen Bellenir. 335 pages. 1999. 0-7808-0327-2. $48.

"This title would be an excellent addition to all public or patient-research libraries." — *American Reference Books Annual, 2001*

"This title is recommended for public, hospital, and health sciences libraries with consumer health collections." — *E-Streams, Jul-Aug '00*

"Recommended reference source." — *Booklist, American Library Association, May '00*

SEE ALSO *Diet & Nutrition Sourcebook, 1st and 2nd Editions, Gastrointestinal Diseases & Disorders Sourcebook*

Disabilities Sourcebook

Basic Consumer Health Information about Physical and Psychiatric Disabilities, Including Descriptions of Major Causes of Disability, Assistive and Adaptive Aids, Workplace Issues, and Accessibility Concerns

Along with Information about the Americans with Disabilities Act, a Glossary, and Resources for Additional Help and Information

Edited by Dawn D. Matthews. 616 pages. 2000. 0-7808-0389-2. $78.

"A much needed addition to the Omnigraphics *Health Reference Series*. A current reference work to provide people with disabilities, their families, caregivers or those who work with them, a broad range of information in one volume, has not been available until now. . . . It is recommended for all public and academic library reference collections." — *E-Streams, May '01*

■

Domestic Violence & Child Abuse Sourcebook

Basic Consumer Health Information about Spousal/ Partner, Child, Sibling, Parent, and Elder Abuse, Covering Physical, Emotional, and Sexual Abuse, Teen Dating Violence, and Stalking; Includes Information about Hotlines, Safe Houses, Safety Plans, and Other Resources for Support and Assistance, Community Initiatives, and Reports on Current Directions in Research and Treatment

Along with a Glossary, Sources for Further Reading, and Governmental and Non-Governmental Organizations Contact Information

Edited by Helene Henderson. 1,064 pages. 2000. 0-7808-0235-7. $78.

■

Drug Abuse Sourcebook

Basic Consumer Health Information about Illicit Substances of Abuse and the Diversion of Prescription Medications, Including Depressants, Hallucinogens, Inhalants, Marijuana, Narcotics, Stimulants, and Anabolic Steroids

Along with Facts about Related Health Risks, Treatment Issues, and Substance Abuse Prevention Programs, a Glossary of Terms, Statistical Data, and Directories of Hotline Services, Self-Help Groups, and Organizations Able to Provide Further Information

Edited by Karen Bellenir. 629 pages. 2000. 0-7808-0242-X. $78.

SEE ALSO *Alcoholism Sourcebook, Substance Abuse Sourcebook*

■

Ear, Nose & Throat Disorders Sourcebook

Basic Information about Disorders of the Ears, Nose, Sinus Cavities, Pharynx, and Larynx, Including Ear Infections, Tinnitus, Vestibular Disorders, Allergic and Non-Allergic Rhinitis, Sore Throats, Tonsillitis, and Cancers That Affect the Ears, Nose, Sinuses, and Throat

Along with Reports on Current Research Initiatives, a Glossary of Related Medical Terms, and a Directory of Sources for Further Help and Information

Edited by Karen Bellenir and Linda M. Shin. 576 pages. 1998. 0-7808-0206-3. $78.

■

Eating Disorders Sourcebook

Basic Consumer Health Information about Eating Disorders, Including Information about Anorexia Nervosa, Bulimia Nervosa, Binge Eating, Body Dysmorphic Disorder, Pica, Laxative Abuse, and Night Eating Syndrome

Along with Information about Causes, Adverse Effects, and Treatment and Prevention Issues, and Featuring a Section on Concerns Specific to Children and Adolescents, a Glossary, and Resources for Further Help and Information

Edited by Dawn D. Matthews. 322 pages. 2001. 0-7808-0335-3. $78.

■

Endocrine & Metabolic Disorders Sourcebook

Basic Information for the Layperson about Pancreatic and Insulin-Related Disorders Such as Pancreatitis, Diabetes, and Hypoglycemia; Adrenal Gland Disorders Such as Cushing's Syndrome, Addison's Disease, and Congenital Adrenal Hyperplasia; Pituitary Gland Disorders Such as Growth Hormone Deficiency, Acromegaly, and Pituitary Tumors; Thyroid Disorders Such as Hypothyroidism, Graves' Disease, Hashimoto's Disease, and Goiter; Hyperparathyroidism; and Other Diseases and Syndromes of Hormone Imbalance or Metabolic Dysfunction

Along with Reports on Current Research Initiatives

Edited by Linda M. Shin. 574 pages. 1998. 0-7808-0207-1. $78.

348

■

Environmentally Induced Disorders Sourcebook

Basic Information about Diseases and Syndromes Linked to Exposure to Pollutants and Other Substances in Outdoor and Indoor Environments Such as Lead, Asbestos, Formaldehyde, Mercury, Emissions, Noise, and More

Edited by Allan R. Cook. 620 pages. 1997. 0-7808-0083-4. $78.

"Recommended reference source."
—*Booklist, American Library Association, Sep '98*

"This book will be a useful addition to anyone's library."
—*Choice Health Sciences Supplement, Association of College and Research Libraries, May '98*

". . . a good survey of numerous environmentally induced physical disorders . . . a useful addition to anyone's library."
—*Doody's Health Sciences Book Reviews, Jan '98*

". . . provide[s] introductory information from the best authorities around. Since this volume covers topics that potentially affect everyone, it will surely be one of the most frequently consulted volumes in the *Health Reference Series*."
—*Rettig on Reference, Nov '97*

■

Ethnic Diseases Sourcebook

Basic Consumer Health Information for Ethnic and Racial Minority Groups in the United States, Including General Health Indicators and Behaviors, Ethnic Diseases, Genetic Testing, the Impact of Chronic Diseases, Women's Health, Mental Health Issues, and Preventive Health Care Services

Along with a Glossary and a Listing of Additional Resources

Edited by Joyce Brennfleck Shannon. 664 pages. 2001. 0-7808-0336-1. $78.

■

Family Planning Sourcebook

Basic Consumer Health Information about Planning for Pregnancy and Contraception, Including Traditional Methods, Barrier Methods, Hormonal Methods, Permanent Methods, Future Methods, Emergency Contraception, and Birth Control Choices for Women at Each Stage of Life

Along with Statistics, a Glossary, and Sources of Additional Information

Edited by Amy Marcaccio Keyzer. 520 pages. 2001. 0-7808-0379-5. $78.

SEE ALSO Pregnancy & Birth Sourcebook

Fitness & Exercise Sourcebook, 1st Edition

Basic Information on Fitness and Exercise, Including Fitness Activities for Specific Age Groups, Exercise for People with Specific Medical Conditions, How to Begin a Fitness Program in Running, Walking, Swimming, Cycling, and Other Athletic Activities, and Recent Research in Fitness and Exercise

Edited by Dan R. Harris. 663 pages. 1996. 0-7808-0186-5. $78.

"A good resource for general readers."
—*Choice, Association of College and Research Libraries, Nov '97*

"The perennial popularity of the topic . . . make this an appealing selection for public libraries."
—*Rettig on Reference, Jun/Jul '97*

■

Fitness & Exercise Sourcebook, 2nd Edition

Basic Consumer Health Information about the Fundamentals of Fitness and Exercise, Including How to Begin and Maintain a Fitness Program, Fitness as a Lifestyle, the Link between Fitness and Diet, Advice for Specific Groups of People, Exercise as It Relates to Specific Medical Conditions, and Recent Research in Fitness and Exercise

Along with a Glossary of Important Terms and Resources for Additional Help and Information

Edited by Kristen M. Gledhill. 646 pages. 2001. 0-7808-0334-5. $78.

■

Food & Animal Borne Diseases Sourcebook

Basic Information about Diseases That Can Be Spread to Humans through the Ingestion of Contaminated Food or Water or by Contact with Infected Animals and Insects, Such as Botulism, E. Coli, Hepatitis A, Trichinosis, Lyme Disease, and Rabies

Along with Information Regarding Prevention and Treatment Methods, and Including a Special Section for International Travelers Describing Diseases Such as Cholera, Malaria, Travelers' Diarrhea, and Yellow Fever, and Offering Recommendations for Avoiding Illness

Edited by Karen Bellenir and Peter D. Dresser. 535 pages. 1995. 0-7808-0033-8. $78.

"Targeting general readers and providing them with a single, comprehensive source of information on selected topics, this book continues, with the excellent caliber of its predecessors, to catalog topical information on health matters of general interest. Readable and thorough, this valuable resource is highly recommended for all libraries."
—*Academic Library Book Review, Summer '96*

"A comprehensive collection of authoritative information."
—*Emergency Medical Services, Oct '95*

Food Safety Sourcebook

Basic Consumer Health Information about the Safe Handling of Meat, Poultry, Seafood, Eggs, Fruit Juices, and Other Food Items, and Facts about Pesticides, Drinking Water, Food Safety Overseas, and the Onset, Duration, and Symptoms of Foodborne Illnesses, Including Types of Pathogenic Bacteria, Parasitic Protozoa, Worms, Viruses, and Natural Toxins

Along with the Role of the Consumer, the Food Handler, and the Government in Food Safety; a Glossary, and Resources for Additional Help and Information

Edited by Dawn D. Matthews. 339 pages. 1999. 0-7808-0326-4. $48.

"This book is recommended for public libraries and universities with home economic and food science programs." — E-Streams, Nov '00

"This book takes the complex issues of food safety and foodborne pathogens and presents them in an easily understood manner. [It does] an excellent job of covering a large and often confusing topic."
—*American Reference Books Annual, 2000*

"Recommended reference source."
—*Booklist, American Library Association, May '00*

■

Forensic Medicine Sourcebook

Basic Consumer Information for the Layperson about Forensic Medicine, Including Crime Scene Investigation, Evidence Collection and Analysis, Expert Testimony, Computer-Aided Criminal Identification, Digital Imaging in the Courtroom, DNA Profiling, Accident Reconstruction, Autopsies, Ballistics, Drugs and Explosives Detection, Latent Fingerprints, Product Tampering, and Questioned Document Examination

Along with Statistical Data, a Glossary of Forensics Terminology, and Listings of Sources for Further Help and Information

Edited by Annemarie S. Muth. 574 pages. 1999. 0-7808-0232-2. $78.

"Given the expected widespread interest in its content and its easy to read style, this book is recommended for most public and all college and university libraries." — E-Streams, Feb '01

"There are several items that make this book attractive to consumers who are seeking certain forensic data. . . . This is a useful current source for those seeking general forensic medical answers."
—*American Reference Books Annual, 2000*

"Recommended for public libraries."
—*Reference & User Services Quarterly, American Library Association, Spring 2000*

"Recommended reference source."
—*Booklist, American Library Association, Feb '00*

"A wealth of information, useful statistics, references are up-to-date and extremely complete. This wonderful collection of data will help students who are interested in a career in any type of forensic field. It is a great

resource for attorneys who need information about types of expert witnesses needed in a particular case. It also offers useful information for fiction and nonfiction writers whose work involves a crime. A fascinating compilation. All levels." — *Choice, Association of College and Research Libraries, Jan 2000*

■

Gastrointestinal Diseases & Disorders Sourcebook

Basic Information about Gastroesophageal Reflux Disease (Heartburn), Ulcers, Diverticulosis, Irritable Bowel Syndrome, Crohn's Disease, Ulcerative Colitis, Diarrhea, Constipation, Lactose Intolerance, Hemorrhoids, Hepatitis, Cirrhosis, and Other Digestive Problems, Featuring Statistics, Descriptions of Symptoms, and Current Treatment Methods of Interest for Persons Living with Upper and Lower Gastrointestinal Maladies

Edited by Linda M. Ross. 413 pages. 1996. 0-7808-0078-8. $78.

". . . very readable form. The successful editorial work that brought this material together into a useful and understandable reference makes accessible to all readers information that can help them more effectively understand and obtain help for digestive tract problems."
— *Choice, Association of College and Research Libraries, Feb '97*

SEE ALSO *Diet & Nutrition Sourcebook, 1st and 2nd Editions, Digestive Diseases & Disorders Sourcebook*

■

Genetic Disorders Sourcebook, 1st Edition

Basic Information about Heritable Diseases and Disorders Such as Down Syndrome, PKU, Hemophilia, Von Willebrand Disease, Gaucher Disease, Tay-Sachs Disease, and Sickle-Cell Disease, Along with Information about Genetic Screening, Gene Therapy, Home Care, and Including Source Listings for Further Help and Information on More Than 300 Disorders

Edited by Karen Bellenir. 642 pages. 1996. 0-7808-0034-6. $78.

"Recommended for undergraduate libraries or libraries that serve the public."
— *Science & Technology Libraries, Vol. 18, No. 1, '99*

"Provides essential medical information to both the general public and those diagnosed with a serious or fatal genetic disease or disorder."
—*Choice, Association of College and Research Libraries, Jan '97*

"Geared toward the lay public. It would be well placed in all public libraries and in those hospital and medical libraries in which access to genetic references is limited." —*Doody's Health Sciences Book Review, Oct '96*

Genetic Disorders Sourcebook, 2nd Edition

Basic Consumer Health Information about Hereditary Diseases and Disorders, Including Cystic Fibrosis, Down Syndrome, Hemophilia, Huntington's Disease, Sickle Cell Anemia, and More; Facts about Genes, Gene Research and Therapy, Genetic Screening, Ethics of Gene Testing, Genetic Counseling, and Advice on Coping and Caring

Along with a Glossary of Genetic Terminology and a Resource List for Help, Support, and Further Information

Edited by Kathy Massimini. 768 pages. 2001. 0-7808-0241-1. $78.

"Recommended for public libraries and medical and hospital libraries with consumer health collections."
— *E-Streams, May '01*

"Recommended reference source."
— *Booklist, American Library Association, Apr '01*

"Important pick for college-level health reference libraries." — *The Bookwatch, Mar '01*

■

Head Trauma Sourcebook

Basic Information for the Layperson about Open-Head and Closed-Head Injuries, Treatment Advances, Recovery, and Rehabilitation

Along with Reports on Current Research Initiatives

Edited by Karen Bellenir. 414 pages. 1997. 0-7808-0208-X. $78.

■

Health Insurance Sourcebook

Basic Information about Managed Care Organizations, Traditional Fee-for-Service Insurance, Insurance Portability and Pre-Existing Conditions Clauses, Medicare, Medicaid, Social Security, and Military Health Care

Along with Information about Insurance Fraud

Edited by Wendy Wilcox. 530 pages. 1997. 0-7808-0222-5. $78.

"Particularly useful because it brings much of this information together in one volume. This book will be a handy reference source in the health sciences library, hospital library, college and university library, and medium to large public library."
— *Medical Reference Services Quarterly, Fall '98*

Awarded "Books of the Year Award"
— *American Journal of Nursing, 1997*

"The layout of the book is particularly helpful as it provides easy access to reference material. A most useful addition to the vast amount of information about health insurance. The use of data from U.S. government agencies is most commendable. Useful in a library or learning center for healthcare professional students."
— *Doody's Health Sciences Book Reviews, Nov '97*

Health Reference Series Cumulative Index 1999

A Comprehensive Index to the Individual Volumes of the Health Reference Series, Including a Subject Index, Name Index, Organization Index, and Publication Index

Along with a Master List of Acronyms and Abbreviations

Edited by Edward J. Prucha, Anne Holmes, and Robert Rudnick. 990 pages. 2000. 0-7808-0382-5. $78.

"This volume will be most helpful in libraries that have a relatively complete collection of the Health Reference Series."
— *American Reference Books Annual, 2001*

"Essential for collections that hold any of the numerous *Health Reference Series* titles."
— *Choice, Association of College and Research Libraries, Nov '00*

■

Healthy Aging Sourcebook

Basic Consumer Health Information about Maintaining Health through the Aging Process, Including Advice on Nutrition, Exercise, and Sleep, Help in Making Decisions about Midlife Issues and Retirement, and Guidance Concerning Practical and Informed Choices in Health Consumerism

Along with Data Concerning the Theories of Aging, Different Experiences in Aging by Minority Groups, and Facts about Aging Now and Aging in the Future; and Featuring a Glossary, a Guide to Consumer Help, Additional Suggested Reading, and Practical Resource Directory

Edited by Jenifer Swanson. 536 pages. 1999. 0-7808-0390-6. $78.

"Recommended reference source."
— *Booklist, American Library Association, Feb '00*

SEE ALSO *Physical & Mental Issues in Aging Sourcebook*

■

Healthy Heart Sourcebook for Women

Basic Consumer Health Information about Cardiac Issues Specific to Women, Including Facts about Major Risk Factors and Prevention, Treatment and Control Strategies, and Important Dietary Issues

Along with a Special Section Regarding the Pros and Cons of Hormone Replacement Therapy and Its Impact on Heart Health, and Additional Help, Including Recipes, a Glossary, and a Directory of Resources

Edited by Dawn D. Matthews. 336 pages. 2000. 0-7808-0329-9. $48.

"A good reference source and recommended for all public, academic, medical, and hospital libraries."
— *Medical Reference Services Quarterly, Summer '01*

"Because of the lack of information specific to women on this topic, this book is recommended for public libraries and consumer libraries."
—American Reference Books Annual, 2001

"Contains very important information about coronary artery disease that all women should know. The information is current and presented in an easy-to-read format. The book will make a good addition to any library." *—American Medical Writers Association Journal, Summer '00*

"Important, basic reference."
—Reviewer's Bookwatch, Jul '00

SEE ALSO *Cardiovascular Diseases & Disorders Sourcebook, 1st Edition, Heart Diseases & Disorders Sourcebook, 2nd Edition, Women's Health Concerns Sourcebook*

■

Heart Diseases & Disorders Sourcebook, 2nd Edition

Basic Consumer Health Information about Heart Attacks, Angina, Rhythm Disorders, Heart Failure, Valve Disease, Congenital Heart Disorders, and More, Including Descriptions of Surgical Procedures and Other Interventions, Medications, Cardiac Rehabilitation, Risk Identification, and Prevention Tips

Along with Statistical Data, Reports on Current Research Initiatives, a Glossary of Cardiovascular Terms, and Resource Directory

Edited by Karen Bellenir. 612 pages. 2000. 0-7808-0238-1. $78.

"This work stands out as an imminently accessible resource for the general public. It is recommended for the reference and circulating shelves of school, public, and academic libraries."
—American Reference Books Annual, 2001

"Recommended reference source."
—Booklist, American Library Association, Dec '00

"Provides comprehensive coverage of matters related to the heart. This title is recommended for health sciences and public libraries with consumer health collections."
—E-Streams, Oct '00

SEE ALSO *Cardiovascular Diseases & Disorders Sourcebook, 1st Edition, Healthy Heart Sourcebook for Women*

■

Immune System Disorders Sourcebook

Basic Information about Lupus, Multiple Sclerosis, Guillain-Barré Syndrome, Chronic Granulomatous Disease, and More

Along with Statistical and Demographic Data and Reports on Current Research Initiatives

Edited by Allan R. Cook. 608 pages. 1997. 0-7808-0209-8. $78.

Infant & Toddler Health Sourcebook

Basic Consumer Health Information about the Physical and Mental Development of Newborns, Infants, and Toddlers, Including Neonatal Concerns, Nutrition Recommendations, Immunization Schedules, Common Pediatric Disorders, Assessments and Milestones, Safety Tips, and Advice for Parents and Other Caregivers

Along with a Glossary of Terms and Resource Listings for Additional Help

Edited by Jenifer Swanson. 585 pages. 2000. 0-7808-0246-2. $78.

"As a reference for the general public, this would be useful in any library." *—E-Streams, May '01*

"Recommended reference source."
—Booklist, American Library Association, Feb '01

"This is a good source for general use."
—American Reference Books Annual, 2001

■

Kidney & Urinary Tract Diseases & Disorders Sourcebook

Basic Information about Kidney Stones, Urinary Incontinence, Bladder Disease, End Stage Renal Disease, Dialysis, and More

Along with Statistical and Demographic Data and Reports on Current Research Initiatives

Edited by Linda M. Ross. 602 pages. 1997. 0-7808-0079-6. $78.

■

Learning Disabilities Sourcebook

Basic Information about Disorders Such as Dyslexia, Visual and Auditory Processing Deficits, Attention Deficit/Hyperactivity Disorder, and Autism

Along with Statistical and Demographic Data, Reports on Current Research Initiatives, an Explanation of the Assessment Process, and a Special Section for Adults with Learning Disabilities

Edited by Linda M. Shin. 579 pages. 1998. 0-7808-0210-1. $78.

Named "Outstanding Reference Book of 1999."
—New York Public Library, Feb 2000

"An excellent candidate for inclusion in a public library reference section. It's a great source of information. Teachers will also find the book useful. Definitely worth reading."
—Journal of Adolescent & Adult Literacy, Feb 2000

"Readable . . . provides a solid base of information regarding successful techniques used with individuals who have learning disabilities, as well as practical suggestions for educators and family members. Clear language, concise descriptions, and pertinent information for contacting multiple resources add to the strength of this book as a useful tool." —*Choice, Association of College and Research Libraries, Feb '99*

"Recommended reference source."
—*Booklist, American Library Association, Sep '98*

"This is a useful resource for libraries and for those who don't have the time to identify and locate the individual publications."
—*Disability Resources Monthly, Sep '98*

■

Liver Disorders Sourcebook

Basic Consumer Health Information about the Liver and How It Works; Liver Diseases, Including Cancer, Cirrhosis, Hepatitis, and Toxic and Drug Related Diseases; Tips for Maintaining a Healthy Liver; Laboratory Tests, Radiology Tests, and Facts about Liver Transplantation

Along with a Section on Support Groups, a Glossary, and Resource Listings

Edited by Joyce Brennfleck Shannon. 591 pages. 2000. 0-7808-0383-3. $78.

"A valuable resource."
—*American Reference Books Annual, 2001*

"This title is recommended for health sciences and public libraries with consumer health collections."
—*E-Streams, Oct '00*

"Recommended reference source."
—*Booklist, American Library Association, Jun '00*

■

Medical Tests Sourcebook

Basic Consumer Health Information about Medical Tests, Including Periodic Health Exams, General Screening Tests, Tests You Can Do at Home, Findings of the U.S. Preventive Services Task Force, X-ray and Radiology Tests, Electrical Tests, Tests of Blood and Other Body Fluids and Tissues, Scope Tests, Lung Tests, Genetic Tests, Pregnancy Tests, Newborn Screening Tests, Sexually Transmitted Disease Tests, and Computer Aided Diagnoses

Along with a Section on Paying for Medical Tests, a Glossary, and Resource Listings

Edited by Joyce Brennfleck Shannon. 691 pages. 1999. 0-7808-0243-8. $78.

"A valuable reference guide."
—*American Reference Books Annual, 2000*

"Recommended for hospital and health sciences libraries with consumer health collections."
—*E-Streams, Mar '00*

"This is an overall excellent reference with a wealth of general knowledge that may aid those who are reluctant to get vital tests performed."
—*Today's Librarian, Jan 2000*

Men's Health Concerns Sourcebook

Basic Information about Health Issues That Affect Men, Featuring Facts about the Top Causes of Death in Men, Including Heart Disease, Stroke, Cancers, Prostate Disorders, Chronic Obstructive Pulmonary Disease, Pneumonia and Influenza, Human Immunodeficiency Virus and Acquired Immune Deficiency Syndrome, Diabetes Mellitus, Stress, Suicide, Accidents and Homicides; and Facts about Common Concerns for Men, Including Impotence, Contraception, Circumcision, Sleep Disorders, Snoring, Hair Loss, Diet, Nutrition, Exercise, Kidney and Urological Disorders, and Backaches

Edited by Allan R. Cook. 738 pages. 1998. 0-7808-0212-8. $78.

"This comprehensive resource and the series are highly recommended."
—*American Reference Books Annual, 2000*

"Recommended reference source."
—*Booklist, American Library Association, Dec '98*

■

Mental Health Disorders Sourcebook, 1st Edition

Basic Information about Schizophrenia, Depression, Bipolar Disorder, Panic Disorder, Obsessive-Compulsive Disorder, Phobias and Other Anxiety Disorders, Paranoia and Other Personality Disorders, Eating Disorders, and Sleep Disorders

Along with Information about Treatment and Therapies

Edited by Karen Bellenir. 548 pages. 1995. 0-7808-0040-0. $78.

"This is an excellent new book . . . written in easy-to-understand language."
—*Booklist Health Sciences Supplement, American Library Association, Oct '97*

". . . useful for public and academic libraries and consumer health collections."
—*Medical Reference Services Quarterly, Spring '97*

"The great strengths of the book are its readability and its inclusion of places to find more information. Especially recommended." —*Reference Quarterly, American Library Association, Winter '96*

". . . a good resource for a consumer health library."
—*Bulletin of the Medical Library Association, Oct '96*

"The information is data-based and couched in brief, concise language that avoids jargon. . . . a useful reference source." —*Readings, Sep '96*

"The text is well organized and adequately written for its target audience." —*Choice, Association of College and Research Libraries, Jun '96*

". . . provides information on a wide range of mental disorders, presented in nontechnical language."
—*Exceptional Child Education Resources, Spring '96*

"Recommended for public and academic libraries."
—*Reference Book Review, 1996*

Mental Health Disorders Sourcebook, 2nd Edition

Basic Consumer Health Information about Anxiety Disorders, Depression and Other Mood Disorders, Eating Disorders, Personality Disorders, Schizophrenia, and More, Including Disease Descriptions, Treatment Options, and Reports on Current Research Initiatives

Along with Statistical Data, Tips for Maintaining Mental Health, a Glossary, and Directory of Sources for Additional Help and Information

Edited by Karen Bellenir. 605 pages. 2000. 0-7808-0240-3. $78.

"Well organized and well written."
—American Reference Books Annual, 2001

"Recommended reference source."
—Booklist, American Library Association, Jun '00

∎

Mental Retardation Sourcebook

Basic Consumer Health Information about Mental Retardation and Its Causes, Including Down Syndrome, Fetal Alcohol Syndrome, Fragile X Syndrome, Genetic Conditions, Injury, and Environmental Sources

Along with Preventive Strategies, Parenting Issues, Educational Implications, Health Care Needs, Employment and Economic Matters, Legal Issues, a Glossary, and a Resource Listing for Additional Help and Information

Edited by Joyce Brennfleck Shannon. 642 pages. 2000. 0-7808-0377-9. $78.

"Public libraries will find the book useful for reference and as a beginning research point for students, parents, and caregivers."
—American Reference Books Annual, 2001

"The strength of this work is that it compiles many basic fact sheets and addresses for further information in one volume. It is intended and suitable for the general public. The sourcebook is relevant to any collection providing health information to the general public."
— E-Streams, Nov '00

"From preventing retardation to parenting and family challenges, this covers health, social and legal issues and will prove an invaluable overview."
— Reviewer's Bookwatch, Jul '00

∎

Obesity Sourcebook

Basic Consumer Health Information about Diseases and Other Problems Associated with Obesity, and Including Facts about Risk Factors, Prevention Issues, and Management Approaches

Along with Statistical and Demographic Data, Information about Special Populations, Research Updates, a Glossary, and Source Listings for Further Help and Information

Edited by Wilma Caldwell and Chad T. Kimball. 376 pages. 2001. 0-7808-0333-7. $48.

" Recommended pick both for specialty health library collections and any general consumer health reference collection." *— The Bookwatch, Apr '01*

"Recommended reference source."
—Booklist, American Library Association, Apr '01

∎

Ophthalmic Disorders Sourcebook

Basic Information about Glaucoma, Cataracts, Macular Degeneration, Strabismus, Refractive Disorders, and More

Along with Statistical and Demographic Data and Reports on Current Research Initiatives

Edited by Linda M. Ross. 631 pages. 1996. 0-7808-0081-8. $78.

∎

Oral Health Sourcebook

Basic Information about Diseases and Conditions Affecting Oral Health, Including Cavities, Gum Disease, Dry Mouth, Oral Cancers, Fever Blisters, Canker Sores, Oral Thrush, Bad Breath, Temporomandibular Disorders, and other Craniofacial Syndromes

Along with Statistical Data on the Oral Health of Americans, Oral Hygiene, Emergency First Aid, Information on Treatment Procedures and Methods of Replacing Lost Teeth

Edited by Allan R. Cook. 558 pages. 1997. 0-7808-0082-6. $78.

"Unique source which will fill a gap in dental sources for patients and the lay public. A valuable reference tool even in a library with thousands of books on dentistry. Comprehensive, clear, inexpensive, and easy to read and use. It fills an enormous gap in the health care literature." *— Reference and User Services Quarterly, American Library Association, Summer '98*

"Recommended reference source."
— Booklist, American Library Association, Dec '97

∎

Osteoporosis Sourcebook

Basic Consumer Health Information about Primary and Secondary Osteoporosis and Juvenile Osteoporosis and Related Conditions, Including Fibrous Dysplasia, Gaucher Disease, Hyperthyroidism, Hypophosphatasia, Myeloma, Osteopetrosis, Osteogenesis Imperfecta, and Paget's Disease

Along with Information about Risk Factors, Treatments, Traditional and Non-Traditional Pain Management, a Glossary of Related Terms, and a Directory of Resources

Edited by Allan R. Cook. 584 pages. 2001. 0-7808-0239-X. $78.

SEE ALSO *Women's Health Concerns Sourcebook*

Pain Sourcebook

Basic Information about Specific Forms of Acute and Chronic Pain, Including Headaches, Back Pain, Muscular Pain, Neuralgia, Surgical Pain, and Cancer Pain

Along with Pain Relief Options Such as Analgesics, Narcotics, Nerve Blocks, Transcutaneous Nerve Stimulation, and Alternative Forms of Pain Control, Including Biofeedback, Imaging, Behavior Modification, and Relaxation Techniques

Edited by Allan R. Cook. 667 pages. 1997. 0-7808-0213-6. $78.

"The text is readable, easily understood, and well indexed. This excellent volume belongs in all patient education libraries, consumer health sections of public libraries, and many personal collections."
— *American Reference Books Annual, 1999*

"A beneficial reference." — *Booklist Health Sciences Supplement, American Library Association, Oct '98*

"The information is basic in terms of scholarship and is appropriate for general readers. Written in journalistic style... intended for non-professionals. Quite thorough in its coverage of different pain conditions and summarizes the latest clinical information regarding pain treatment." — *Choice, Association of College and Research Libraries, Jun '98*

"Recommended reference source."
— *Booklist, American Library Association, Mar '98*

Pediatric Cancer Sourcebook

Basic Consumer Health Information about Leukemias, Brain Tumors, Sarcomas, Lymphomas, and Other Cancers in Infants, Children, and Adolescents, Including Descriptions of Cancers, Treatments, and Coping Strategies

Along with Suggestions for Parents, Caregivers, and Concerned Relatives, a Glossary of Cancer Terms, and Resource Listings

Edited by Edward J. Prucha. 587 pages. 1999. 0-7808-0245-4. $78.

"A valuable addition to all libraries specializing in health services and many public libraries."
— *American Reference Books Annual, 2000*

"Recommended reference source."
— *Booklist, American Library Association, Feb '00*

"An excellent source of information. Recommended for public, hospital, and health science libraries with consumer health collections." — *E-Streams, Jun '00*

Physical & Mental Issues in Aging Sourcebook

Basic Consumer Health Information on Physical and Mental Disorders Associated with the Aging Process, Including Concerns about Cardiovascular Disease, Pulmonary Disease, Oral Health, Digestive Disorders, Musculoskeletal and Skin Disorders, Metabolic Changes, Sexual and Reproductive Issues, and Changes in Vision, Hearing, and Other Senses

Along with Data about Longevity and Causes of Death, Information on Acute and Chronic Pain, Descriptions of Mental Concerns, a Glossary of Terms, and Resource Listings for Additional Help

Edited by Jenifer Swanson. 660 pages. 1999. 0-7808-0233-0. $78.

"Recommended for public libraries."
— *American Reference Books Annual, 2000*

"This is a treasure of health information for the layperson." — *Choice Health Sciences Supplement, Association of College & Research Libraries, May 2000*

"Recommended reference source."
— *Booklist, American Library Association, Oct '99*

SEE ALSO Healthy Aging Sourcebook

Podiatry Sourcebook

Basic Consumer Health Information about Foot Conditions, Diseases, and Injuries, Including Bunions, Corns, Calluses, Athlete's Foot, Plantar Warts, Hammertoes and Clawtoes, Clubfoot, Heel Pain, Gout, and More

Along with Facts about Foot Care, Disease Prevention, Foot Safety, Choosing a Foot Care Specialist, a Glossary of Terms, and Resource Listings for Additional Information

Edited by M. Lisa Weatherford. 400 pages. 2001. 0-7808-0215-2. $78.

Pregnancy & Birth Sourcebook

Basic Information about Planning for Pregnancy, Maternal Health, Fetal Growth and Development, Labor and Delivery, Postpartum and Perinatal Care, Pregnancy in Mothers with Special Concerns, and Disorders of Pregnancy, Including Genetic Counseling, Nutrition and Exercise, Obstetrical Tests, Pregnancy Discomfort, Multiple Births, Cesarean Sections, Medical Testing of Newborns, Breastfeeding, Gestational Diabetes, and Ectopic Pregnancy

Edited by Heather E. Aldred. 737 pages. 1997. 0-7808-0216-0. $78.

"A well-organized handbook. Recommended."
— *Choice, Association of College and Research Libraries, Apr '98*

"Recommended reference source."
— *Booklist, American Library Association, Mar '98*

"Recommended for public libraries."
— *American Reference Books Annual, 1998*

SEE ALSO Congenital Disorders Sourcebook, Family Planning Sourcebook

Prostate Cancer Sourcebook

Basic Consumer Health Information about Prostate Cancer, Including Information about the Associated Risk Factors, Detection, Diagnosis, and Treatment of Prostate Cancer

Along with Information on Non-Malignant Prostate Conditions, and Featuring a Section Listing Support and Treatment Centers and a Glossary of Related Terms

Edited by Dawn D. Matthews. 358 pages. 2001. 0-7808-0324-8. $78.

■

Public Health Sourcebook

Basic Information about Government Health Agencies, Including National Health Statistics and Trends, Healthy People 2000 Program Goals and Objectives, the Centers for Disease Control and Prevention, the Food and Drug Administration, and the National Institutes of Health

Along with Full Contact Information for Each Agency

Edited by Wendy Wilcox. 698 pages. 1998. 0-7808-0220-9. $78.

"Recommended reference source."
— *Booklist, American Library Association, Sep '98*

"This consumer guide provides welcome assistance in navigating the maze of federal health agencies and their data on public health concerns."
— *SciTech Book News, Sep '98*

■

Reconstructive & Cosmetic Surgery Sourcebook

Basic Consumer Health Information on Cosmetic and Reconstructive Plastic Surgery, Including Statistical Information about Different Surgical Procedures, Things to Consider Prior to Surgery, Plastic Surgery Techniques and Tools, Emotional and Psychological Considerations, and Procedure-Specific Information

Along with a Glossary of Terms and a Listing of Resources for Additional Help and Information

Edited by M. Lisa Weatherford. 374 pages. 2001. 0-7808-0214-4. $48.

■

Rehabilitation Sourcebook

Basic Consumer Health Information about Rehabilitation for People Recovering from Heart Surgery, Spinal Cord Injury, Stroke, Orthopedic Impairments, Amputation, Pulmonary Impairments, Traumatic Injury, and More, Including Physical Therapy, Occupational Therapy, Speech/ Language Therapy, Massage Therapy, Dance Therapy, Art Therapy, and Recreational Therapy

Along with Information on Assistive and Adaptive Devices, a Glossary, and Resources for Additional Help and Information

Edited by Dawn D. Matthews. 531 pages. 1999. 0-7808-0236-5. $78.

"This is an excellent resource for public library reference and health collections."
— *American Reference Books Annual, 2001*

"Recommended reference source."
— *Booklist, American Library Association, May '00*

■

Respiratory Diseases & Disorders Sourcebook

Basic Information about Respiratory Diseases and Disorders, Including Asthma, Cystic Fibrosis, Pneumonia, the Common Cold, Influenza, and Others, Featuring Facts about the Respiratory System, Statistical and Demographic Data, Treatments, Self-Help Management Suggestions, and Current Research Initiatives

Edited by Allan R. Cook and Peter D. Dresser. 771 pages. 1995. 0-7808-0037-0. $78.

"Designed for the layperson and for patients and their families coping with respiratory illness. . . . an extensive array of information on diagnosis, treatment, management, and prevention of respiratory illnesses for the general reader."
— *Choice, Association of College and Research Libraries, Jun '96*

"A highly recommended text for all collections. It is a comforting reminder of the power of knowledge that good books carry between their covers."
— *Academic Library Book Review, Spring '96*

"A comprehensive collection of authoritative information presented in a nontechnical, humanitarian style for patients, families, and caregivers."
— *Association of Operating Room Nurses, Sep/Oct '95*

■

Sexually Transmitted Diseases Sourcebook, 1st Edition

Basic Information about Herpes, Chlamydia, Gonorrhea, Hepatitis, Nongonoccocal Urethritis, Pelvic Inflammatory Disease, Syphilis, AIDS, and More

Along with Current Data on Treatments and Preventions

Edited by Linda M. Ross. 550 pages. 1997. 0-7808-0217-9. $78.

Sexually Transmitted Diseases Sourcebook, 2nd Edition

Basic Consumer Health Information about Sexually Transmitted Diseases, Including Information on the Diagnosis and Treatment of Chlamydia, Gonorrhea, Hepatitis, Herpes, HIV, Mononucleosis, Syphilis, and Others

Along with Information on Prevention, Such as Condom Use, Vaccines, and STD Education; And Featuring a Section on Issues Related to Youth and Adolescents, a Glossary, and Resources for Additional Help and Information

Edited by Dawn D. Matthews. 538 pages. 2001. 0-7808-0249-7. $78.

"Recommended pick both for specialty health library collections and any general consumer health reference collection." — *The Bookwatch, Apr '01*

"Recommended reference source."
— *Booklist, American Library Association, Apr '01*

■

Skin Disorders Sourcebook

Basic Information about Common Skin and Scalp Conditions Caused by Aging, Allergies, Immune Reactions, Sun Exposure, Infectious Organisms, Parasites, Cosmetics, and Skin Traumas, Including Abrasions, Cuts, and Pressure Sores

Along with Information on Prevention and Treatment

Edited by Allan R. Cook. 647 pages. 1997. 0-7808-0080-X. $78.

". . . comprehensive, easily read reference book."
— *Doody's Health Sciences Book Reviews, Oct '97*

SEE ALSO *Burns Sourcebook*

■

Sleep Disorders Sourcebook

Basic Consumer Health Information about Sleep and Its Disorders, Including Insomnia, Sleepwalking, Sleep Apnea, Restless Leg Syndrome, and Narcolepsy

Along with Data about Shiftwork and Its Effects, Information on the Societal Costs of Sleep Deprivation, Descriptions of Treatment Options, a Glossary of Terms, and Resource Listings for Additional Help

Edited by Jenifer Swanson. 439 pages. 1998. 0-7808-0234-9. $78.

"This text will complement any home or medical library. It is user-friendly and ideal for the adult reader." — *American Reference Books Annual, 2000*

"Recommended reference source."
— *Booklist, American Library Association, Feb '99*

"A useful resource that provides accurate, relevant, and accessible information on sleep to the general public. Health care providers who deal with sleep disorders patients may also find it helpful in being prepared to answer some of the questions patients ask."
— *Respiratory Care, Jul '99*

Sports Injuries Sourcebook

Basic Consumer Health Information about Common Sports Injuries, Prevention of Injury in Specific Sports, Tips for Training, and Rehabilitation from Injury

Along with Information about Special Concerns for Children, Young Girls in Athletic Training Programs, Senior Athletes, and Women Athletes, and a Directory of Resources for Further Help and Information

Edited by Heather E. Aldred. 624 pages. 1999. 0-7808-0218-7. $78.

"Public libraries and undergraduate academic libraries will find this book useful for its nontechnical language." — *American Reference Books Annual, 2000*

"While this easy-to-read book is recommended for all libraries, it should prove to be especially useful for public, high school, and academic libraries; certainly it should be on the bookshelf of every school gymnasium." — *E-Streams, Mar '00*

■

Substance Abuse Sourcebook

Basic Health-Related Information about the Abuse of Legal and Illegal Substances Such as Alcohol, Tobacco, Prescription Drugs, Marijuana, Cocaine, and Heroin; and Including Facts about Substance Abuse Prevention Strategies, Intervention Methods, Treatment and Recovery Programs, and a Section Addressing the Special Problems Related to Substance Abuse during Pregnancy

Edited by Karen Bellenir. 573 pages. 1996. 0-7808-0038-9. $78.

"A valuable addition to any health reference section. Highly recommended."
— *The Book Report, Mar/Apr '97*

". . . a comprehensive collection of substance abuse information that's both highly readable and compact. Families and caregivers of substance abusers will find the information enlightening and helpful, while teachers, social workers and journalists should benefit from the concise format. Recommended."
— *Drug Abuse Update, Winter '96/'97*

SEE ALSO *Alcoholism Sourcebook, Drug Abuse Sourcebook*

■

Transplantation Sourcebook

Basic Consumer Health Information about Organ and Tissue Transplantation, Including Physical and Financial Preparations, Procedures and Issues Relating to Specific Solid Organ and Tissue Transplants, Rehabilitation, Pediatric Transplant Information, the Future of Transplantation, and Organ and Tissue Donation

Along with a Glossary and Listings of Additional Resources

Edited by Joyce Brennfleck Shannon. 600 pages. 2001. 0-7808-0322-1. $78.

Traveler's Health Sourcebook

Basic Consumer Health Information for Travelers, Including Physical and Medical Preparations, Transportation Health and Safety, Essential Information about Food and Water, Sun Exposure, Insect and Snake Bites, Camping and Wilderness Medicine, and Travel with Physical or Medical Disabilities

Along with International Travel Tips, Vaccination Recommendations, Geographical Health Issues, Disease Risks, a Glossary, and a Listing of Additional Resources

Edited by Joyce Brennfleck Shannon. 613 pages. 2000. 0-7808-0384-1. $78.

"Recommended reference source."

— *Booklist, American Library Association, Feb '01*

"This book is recommended for any public library, any travel collection, and especially any collection for the physically disabled."

—*American Reference Books Annual, 2001*

■

Women's Health Concerns Sourcebook

Basic Information about Health Issues That Affect Women, Featuring Facts about Menstruation and Other Gynecological Concerns, Including Endometriosis, Fibroids, Menopause, and Vaginitis; Reproductive Concerns, Including Birth Control, Infertility, and Abortion; and Facts about Additional Physical, Emotional, and Mental Health Concerns Prevalent among Women Such as Osteoporosis, Urinary Tract Disorders, Eating Disorders, and Depression

Along with Tips for Maintaining a Healthy Lifestyle

Edited by Heather E. Aldred. 567 pages. 1997. 0-7808-0219-5. $78.

"Handy compilation. There is an impressive range of diseases, devices, disorders, procedures, and other physical and emotional issues covered . . . well organized, illustrated, and indexed." — *Choice, Association of College and Research Libraries, Jan '98*

SEE ALSO *Breast Cancer Sourcebook, Cancer Sourcebook for Women, 1st and 2nd Editions, Healthy Heart Sourcebook for Women, Osteoporosis Sourcebook*

Workplace Health & Safety Sourcebook

Basic Consumer Health Information about Workplace Health and Safety, Including the Effect of Workplace Hazards on the Lungs, Skin, Heart, Ears, Eyes, Brain, Reproductive Organs, Musculoskeletal System, and Other Organs and Body Parts

Along with Information about Occupational Cancer, Personal Protective Equipment, Toxic and Hazardous Chemicals, Child Labor, Stress, and Workplace Violence

Edited by Chad T. Kimball. 626 pages. 2000. 0-7808-0231-4. $78.

"Provides helpful information for primary care physicians and other caregivers interested in occupational medicine. . . . General readers; professionals."

— *Choice, Association of College and Research Libraries, May '01*

"Recommended reference source."

— *Booklist, American Library Association, Feb '01*

"Highly recommended." —*The Bookwatch, Jan '01*

■

Worldwide Health Sourcebook

Basic Information about Global Health Issues, Including Malnutrition, Reproductive Health, Disease Dispersion and Prevention, Emerging Diseases, Risky Health Behaviors, and the Leading Causes of Death

Along with Global Health Concerns for Children, Women, and the Elderly, Mental Health Issues, Research and Technology Advancements, and Economic, Environmental, and Political Health Implications, a Glossary, and a Resource Listing for Additional Help and Information

Edited by Joyce Brennfleck Shannon. 614 pages. 2001. 0-7808-0330-2. $78.